Deaf in the Body

A deaf man's journey through the hearing world

Kevin Fitzgerald

First published in the UK in 2013 by Kevin Fitzgerald

A CIP catalogue record for this title is available
from the British Library

ISBN: 978-0-9564756-1-9

Typeset by Andrew Searle

Printed and bound in the UK by Heaton Press Ltd

KEVIN FITZGERALD
543 Oldham Road,
Middleton, Manchester, M24 2DH
Email: kevinfitz35@yahoo.co.uk

Contents

Forewords

AS A MANCHESTER boy born and bred, I recall the pleasure of going to see my dad's family and grandmother in Collyhurst and Ancoats. Manchester is a city steeped in history and unique with its heritage and diverse mixture of cultures, one of which is deaf culture, having three deaf clubs all within a few square miles of the city centre. It is with some pride and a smile I write this foreword to Kevin's sequel to *Deafness of the Mind*. Many of us at one time or another in our lives have experienced discrimination, bullying and downright hostile treatment. Our shared and personal experience of oppression and anger have made us what we are today; it honed our political skills and a desire to see equality for all.

We now have legislation that protects us. In the early 1990s we had the Disability Discrimination Act (DDA), which transformed the lives of all deaf and disabled people. We now also have the Equality Act, but back in the 1950s and 60s there was nothing like this, it was everyone for themselves.

Kevin takes us on a journey of trials and tribulations where bullying and discrimination were rife; he takes us on a journey from his time at St John's RC School, Boston Spa to his employment in the building trade, where he fondly reminisces of a bygone world where life and limb was at risk almost at every level of employment. How many of you remember the iconic photograph of those steelworkers sitting on one of the steel girders swinging in the air high up above New York City, USA, where health and safety was not even a byword. Kevin leads us through some lovely anecdotes of those truly wonderful friendships and camaraderie from a bygone age...

I warmly welcome you to read this personal journey from an inspiring man who overcame such adversity and is now enjoying his twilight years with his family and Great grandchildren.

Terry Riley
Deaf activist at heart

IT SEEMS EASY to imagine what it is to be colour blind by simply switching the television in black and white. Similarly, a hearing person may think that simply switching off the sound enables them to imagine what it is like to be deaf. They could not be more wrong. Deafness from an early age is one of the most difficult conditions to understand, and this lack of understanding by others is one of the most handicapping aspects of being deaf. This is why first-hand, credible deaf eye-witness accounts like the following by Kevin Fitzgerald are so important in showing the true circumstances of deaf people in our society, incidentally showing features of that society that many would prefer to ignore and sweep under the carpet. The author shows his Irish descent in the fluency of his narrative and in a characteristically open, outspoken attention to frank detail that suggests more than a dash of the rebel in his make-up. It is honesty liable to make him as many enemies as the charm of his prose style will gain him friends.

The salient features of his life and times are described with a clarity that enables the reader to view what to many will be a completely novel visual world and his empathy with the great Beethoven when cut off from his auditory masterpieces is very enlightening for anyone wishing to understand the deaf condition. Chronologically and logically, a beginning is made by describing the misguided education of deaf children during the time that the doctrine of 'Oralism' was used to justify banning sign language and manual communication in schools for the deaf. The author, while noting that he may be biased, wholeheartedly disapproves of this approach. "My mind boggles at the sheer stupidity of it all," he writes, noting that "I just cannot understand how it was allowed to happen." In fact, his account shows some clueful insights into the psychology of oppressive indoctrination, which explains much. For the defence, much of the oralist dogma in British and Irish schools was influenced by the scholarly work of Father Anthony Van Uden, which originated in Nazi-occupied Netherlands and was designed to make deaf children 'normal' to save them from the death squads.

Kevin gives a rare expression to the sense of freedom and euphoria of school-leaving and wades into life, love and work as a roofer in the days before health and safety and political correctness regulations were enforced. He dwells in a world far removed from many middle class assumptions and describes incidents of raw vitality which are sometimes painfully accurate. Truth and diplomacy rarely go together and, for one so sceptical of science, Kevin has settled for scientific accuracy over the historical conspiracy of silence that is still favoured by many Oralism deniers.

George Montgomery
Deaf History Review

I FIRST MET Kevin in 2003 when I enrolled as a student in his sign language classes in Rochdale. I remember being very nervous on that first day when turning up for class, as I'm sure was the case with the other learners. Learning a new language, especially in such a public setting, can be far more daunting than learning almost any other skill. When the student takes his/her first stumbling steps with a language, he is acutely aware of his inadequacies and the fact that those around who can hear – or in this case see – his/her attempts know this too. However, Kevin put us all at ease the moment he came into the room.

What sets him apart is his ability to tell a good story, and to involve his audience as fully as possible in the telling. Now what you are about to read is not fiction, but a life story retold. This book tells of Kevin's memories of finding his place in the hearing world as a young man and the struggles he faced to prove himself. It is a simple story, but well told. Like any story told many years after the events it describes there are digressions (into commentaries on deaf education and employment discrimination), but these are important and to the point. I remember when Kevin would tell such stories in our sign classes about his time as a roofer, the tales told to him by his friends, as well as the discrimination he faced as a worker at the Royal Mail. However, writing this book has given Kevin the chance to fill in many of the details that got left out when I saw these stories first being re-enacted in our sign classes.

I cannot comment directly on the discrimination that Kevin and other deaf people experience, or whether things are getting better, though I hope they are. With the continued advance of technology, people can now communicate via text or video directly onto their phones (which are now fully-developed pocket computers in terms of what they can do). This means that the kinds of discrimination that Kevin faced with some of his employers is getting harder to hide, now that people can record and share information instantly all over the world. I wonder if Kevin and the other deaf employees at the Royal Mail would have been treated better if they'd had the ability to record and post their experiences on something like Facebook or You Tube? Technologies like these make communication easier between deaf and hearing people. As Kevin suggests in his book and elsewhere, the long-term solution is better education for deaf children, where, if appropriate, they can be taught lessons in sign, as well as learning English grammar as it is written and spoken by the much larger hearing population.

I don't think the BSL (British Sign Language) versus SSE (Sign Supported English) debate is going to go away any time soon. Though the important thing is that the deaf are able to communicate effectively in the hearing world and be able to stand up for themselves. As Kevin's experiences suggest, the solution cannot be to rely on others to break down communication and discrimination barriers. When he left Boston Spa, the institution where he spent the majority of his childhood, signing was rarely understood. Imagine how Kevin must have felt when he began a job in the roofing trade of 1950s Manchester! But, as his book shows, he didn't back down, and kept trying until he was understood and respected by his workmates.

Above all, Kevin's story reminds us that people, young and old, deaf and hearing, often need encouragement so that they can achieve, but only so long as they don't accept the low standards and defeatism that the world expects of them all-too-often.

Kevin's story inspired me not to give up when, due to self-doubt on my part, I was ready to throw in the towel at the university, swallow my pride, and beg for a paying job again at the council. (So I offer you thanks Kev, if only for that!) The point is that whatever hardships he faced, Kevin's experiences and their retelling have made a real difference to the lives of others, and this book is a reflection of that.

Paul Hubbard
A pupil and friend of Kevin's

Author's Preface

THIS IS A story that begs to be told, especially as because of the terrible education that the majority of deaf children had to endure when the oral system of teaching deaf kids was in force, not many deaf people are able to put their thoughts down on paper and so are ignored by society. That is the reason why I have written my two books. I am sure that many people, especially those involved in the church and education, will object to what I have to say, but remember, this is what I as a deaf man have lived through. I am not writing about what some scientists have discovered by research. Read about the mistakes of the past, and make sure those mistakes are not repeated, that is the best way to learn.

In my first book, *Deafness of the Mind*, I told the story of my childhood in Collyhurst, a suburb in North Manchester, and how I lived through the German blitzing of my homet own. I described life in the air raid shelters and the bombed out streets that were our playground. At six years old I contracted meningitis, which left me profoundly deaf. The transition from a world of noise, music and laughter to one of an eerie silence is hard to describe, the whole world had changed, and I was in a strange and alien place and felt so helpless. For the first two years before I was sent away to St John's I clung to my mam like a leech.

I didn't realise it at the time, but becoming deaf had opened up a whole new world to me: my sight became keener, I developed the ability to read lips and also to read facial expressions and body language and somehow I managed to stumble along. Then, one fine September day in 1943, I was sent to St John's Institution for the Deaf and Dumb in Boston Spa, West Yorkshire. Alighting from the bus outside this institution, the kindly nun who had accompanied me from Manchester and myself were confronted by a huge sign with the legend, 'St John's Institution for the Deaf and Dumb'. That demeaning sign wouldn't be allowed in this day, would it?

After the Nun had gone back to Manchester I found I was saying to myself over and over, "She's gone back home and left me. She's gone back home and left me". I was very worried that I would never see my mam and dad, my brother Jimmy, my sister Pat or my Collyhurst pals ever again. Nobody had bothered to explain what was happening to me. Try to imagine yourself waking up into a world where people communicated by just moving their mouths, no sound, sparrows don't chirp anymore, cars are right on top of you before you are aware of them and people are impatient if you don't understand them straight away. Heck! I couldn't even walk straight any more. I certainly was one bewildered little boy.

But *Deafness of the Mind* is not a tale of woe, nor is this sequel. It is a story of a little kid who didn't let his disability get in his way. It may be worth reading just for the inspirational value. To try to step into someone else's shoes, if only through a book, can be a mind enriching experience. It's a story of a kid who lived many years ago, it's about a kid who had determination, a kid who was relentless in his search for answers, a kid who was determined to prove that despite his handicap he was as good, if not better, than the next bloke. A kid that when he got knocked down, got up again, and again and again, and it is about a kid who grew up stronger and could fight for himself in many ways in his journey through life.

From the deaf teacher and scoutmaster, Mr Caproni I had learned how to have confidence in myself and to develop the 'I can do it mindset'. He showed by example that a deaf man can achieve success in life. If you cannot talk, well so what! Let your actions and results do your talking. If people put barriers in front of you, and many will try, find a way round them, obstacles don't have to stop you. If you run into a wall don't just give up and turn around, plan how you can climb over it, go through it or work round it, or even how to knock it down, don't let it stop you. That is what he did, that is what I resolved to do when I left St John's. Don't expect any help from the hearing community and you won't be disappointed. Strive with all your might to become independent.

So make yourself comfy, pour a drink, put your feet up and read about this kid and learn how he handled his deafness and what happened to him in his journey through the hearing world after he left St John's.

Kevin Fitzgerald

Family Man

There is no failure except in no longer trying
Elbert Hubbard

THE 1950s! WHAT a great decade that was to be young and alive. That was the decade that gave birth to space travel and rock and roll and finally saw an end to rationing. Though food and utilities were by no means plentiful yet, we could see the light at the end of the tunnel. King George had died and the new Elizabethan years began in 1952, with Mount Everest conquered at last the following year. It was also the decade when I left St John's Institution for the Deaf and Dumb [sic] in Boston Spa for good. I can't describe the feeling of joy and elation I felt in 1951 to at last be free from that establishment. I have found words such as empyrean or euphoria in the dictionary when searching for suitable words to describe the feeling, but they seem so inadequate when describing the feeling of freedom and being able to make decisions by myself without having to ask anyone's permission; freedom from having my day planned down to the last detail by someone else. Maybe some kids were comfortable with other people having the responsibility of making all their decisions for them as they'd become institutionalised, but I hadn't yet and I hated it. Then I realised that the word I was searching for was there right in front of me - it was FREEDOM; freedom that was so precious that we had just fought and won a war for it.

I also met my future wife Diana Taylor in 1954. I was at a loose end one weekend and feeling bored with nothing to do, so I thought I would drop in at Father Hayward's club and see what was happening. So the next Sunday morning

I caught the bus into town and walked up Deansgate until I came to his church on Chester Road. On entering I was met by Terry Riley, the current BDA (British Deaf Association) chairman's father of the same name. He told me to go into the room on the left and have a look at the beautiful girl there. Then he admonished me not to get too excited, and that I must keep calm and not stare too much or I would frighten her. I thought that he was just being silly, but when I entered the room and saw her I did exactly what he had told me not to do. I stood there gaping at her with my mouth open like an idiot. She was surrounded by people and they were all trying to get her attention. As I was looking at her awestruck, she looked over them towards me and our eyes locked and I nearly fainted. Everything seemed to just melt away. Where the room had been full of people only seconds earlier, it now seemed that they had all disappeared and this lovely girl and I were the only people there.

I knew as soon as I set my eyes on her that she was the girl for me; no one else would do for me now, no other girl could compare. I was spellbound. From that moment I was a big believer in love at first sight. My legs were like rubber but I managed to walk over to her and introduce myself as casually as I could. Inside my heart was pounding. I was glad that they were all deaf and couldn't hear it banging away. She looked coolly at me and said, "I'm pleased to meet you, my name is Diana." I knew that my life would never be the same again. How could it possibly be!

After a short spell of Diana playing hard to get and me trying not to show too much eagerness in case I frightened her away, she agreed to be my girlfriend. Later on I was told that I had angered the priest, who was wont to play matchmaker, and he had Diana earmarked for some other person, but I had upset his plans. I had wondered why he was suddenly unfriendly towards me, and now I knew the reason. I know that it's hard to believe but it was like that in those days, and he had arranged a few such matches. It was called being a 'patriarch' and he thought he could do the same with Diana. But I thought to myself that he had gone too far here and could go to the devil and die. He had come up against a force of nature that wouldn't be denied, and I would fight anybody who said that she wasn't my girl, even a priest, so I would!

In the early 1950s, my wages as a cutter in the clothing trade were £5 10s a week. It was a nice clean job, my hands were soft and my nails were spotless, but on those wages I knew that it would be many many years before I could save up enough to marry Diana. Also, my dad was in hospital. Like many of his generation who didn't know better, he had been a boozer and smoker for most of his life, and his unhealthy lifestyle was catching up with him now. Mum was finding it a struggle managing without dad's wages coming in. I was convinced that I had to find a better paying job, but having left St John's, Institution for the Deaf and Dumb at the age of 16 with no qualifications at all, it wasn't going to be easy. As a single lad in the early 1950s those wages that I was earning were adequate for my needs: beer was only one shilling a pint (that's 5p in today's money). Life was simple in those halcyon days of the early 1950s and my needs were few. It was possible to have a good night out with the lads on less than 10 shillings (50p). So, on the advice of a deaf man named Peter Kilgour, I applied for, and got, a job in the roofing trade as a labourer. The wages that I earned there would enable me to save up enough to ask Diana to be my wife.

We were married on June 27th, 1959, the last year of that magic decade. All those momentous things happened to me in the 1950s, so you can see why that decade was such a great, magical one for me. Our first daughter Rosemary was born on July 13th, 1961; it was a magical event just to see that beautiful little baby that Diana and I had made. My life couldn't get any better. Our second daughter, Lynn, was born on December 8th, 1965, another beautiful little girl. Lynn was a very calm, placid little baby and was a joy to hold and cuddle. Finally, our son John was born on February 1st, 1971, a handsome little boy.

When we got home from the hospital with our little John, all was well at first, but a few days later he began to bring up his milk. He couldn't digest his food as he would feed hungrily, then a few moments later he would spew it all up. Unlike the other two babies John was not gaining any weight. He was, in fact, losing weight. It was very worrying, so, on the advice of the doctor, we changed to bottle feeding him, but it made no difference as he was still bringing it all up again. Back to hospital we went with him. They kept him in hospital and found out there was a blockage in his intestine that was causing the problem, so we signed the consent forms for John to have an operation to clear the blockage. It was a very worrying time because John was such a tiny thing and they were going to cut him open. We seemed to spend all our time praying and worrying. He was such a tiny baby and so helpless, I don't think that we would have been able to cope if we had lost him. We waited for hours in the hospital, then the doctor came and said that the operation was successful and we could take him home in a few days when they were sure that he was alright. Phew! What a relief that was. We went home feeling much better.

Next day when we visited we were informed that John would have to have another operation because the first one had failed and he still couldn't keep his feed down. I thought that I was a tough bloke, but Diana was much stronger than me. I just sat there crying like a big baby, I couldn't help it. After some time the doctor came and told us that it was all over and John was comfortable and we could take him home in a few days. At last we had our John home with us and then his weight began to shoot up and soon he was a happy, chubby little baby. I thought it was amazing how the doctors could operate successfully on such a little baby. Our John is now a massive 16-stone strong man. He still has that horrible scar across his stomach to this day, but that is a badge of honour now

I have never ceased to be amazed by how Diana took to motherhood. To see how she handled our kids was amazing, everything just seemed to come naturally to her, her deafness didn't matter at all. There were none of the gadgets that modern day mums have to help them to manage. Things like intercoms to let them know if a baby was crying were no use to Diana. She had her own methods. For example, she would make sure that the baby's cot was touching our bed and if the baby was restless during the night then Diana knew by feeling the vibrations the cot made against the foot of our bed.

Early one Saturday morning Diana nudged me awake with her elbow and gestured for me to be quiet, then she pointed to the cot at the bottom of the bed. I looked and Rosemary, who was just starting to crawl, was waving her legs in the air. Then she tried to stand up in her cot, holding on to the bars as we lay there quietly watching. She managed to stand up, then she put one leg over the top of her cot, pulling herself up and rolling over onto our bed as we watched spellbound. She crawled up and got into bed between Diana and me and then she did a wee in the bed, got out again and started to crawl back to her own little cot. We jumped out of bed, Diana expertly changing her nappy, tucking her up in her cot again and giving her the comfort cloth that helped her to sleep, so thumb in mouth and holding tight to her comfort cloth Rosemary was soon fast asleep again.

I thought that I was the luckiest man in the world. Diana was so beautiful. She had an inner beauty too; she was just like a deaf 'Snow White'. I was truly smitten, even little animals, stray dogs, cats, donkeys and sheep in the nearby field seemed to gravitate towards her. I never thought it was possible to feel like this about another person. I vowed to start going to church again to give thanks to God for making my life so beautiful.

At the time I was playing football for the Salford Deaf Club on Quay St, off Deansgate in Manchester and not far from Father Hayward's small club. The Salford Deaf Club was in a big old rambling Victorian house next to the Opera House. There were lots of nooks and crannies and many small and big rooms, billiard tables, darts, table tennis etc. My deaf friend Peter Kilgour had taken me there and introduced me to everybody. Mr Telling was the social worker who looked after the place. He was a father figure to the deaf people who went there and sorted out any problems they had. As well as football, there was cricket, billiards, snooker, darts etc. We had a very good social life. We were in the Chorlton Amateur Football League and we had our home ground at Hough End playing fields near Southern Cemetery in Chorlton. We also competed in the British Deaf North West Sports leagues and travelled some distances to play deaf clubs in Liverpool, Preston, Warrington etc.

Strangely, I don't remember much about the wet, cold, miserable, windy days playing football with the freezing wind whistling around my frost-bitten knees, I only remember the fine, sunny days when I really enjoyed playing. The worst game I can remember had nothing to do with the weather, but the memory has stayed with me to this day. It was playing football on a field in Newton Heath. Instead of grass the field was covered in crushed red-brick shale, and some of the pieces of crushed brick had very sharp edges. The scrapes and abrasions we had on our knees and elbows soon taught us to be very careful how we tackled. There were no sliding tackles on that field, unless you didn't mind scraping the skin off your legs and elbows. We couldn't play with normal studs on our boots, it was too painful, the ground was too hard for studs. It was like playing on concrete that was covered with rough sandpaper, so we had to take the studs off and put leather bars on which were easier on our feet when playing on that hard red shale.

There were quite a few fields in north Manchester that were covered in this red-brick shale, quite a few footballers who played on those 'Red Recs' were later to turn professional. I know that Bert Trautmann, the Manchester City goalkeeping legend was one of them. Peter Kilgour was asked to have a trial at City, but when he went to see what it was like, after thinking about it he declined the offer because he said all the hearing players were shouting to each other 'pass the ball' or 'over here' and in the dressing room he was ignored by the other players. He felt excluded and he knew that he would be left out, so he decided that it wasn't for him. I knew from past experiences that these hearing players didn't mean to ignore him like that; they were just not deaf aware. They didn't know how to approach him and communicate with him, but he said he would rather stick with his deaf mates, he felt more comfortable with them.

The Corporation got that crushed brick shale in truckloads from the local brick works on Barney's Croft, which was situated just off Queens Road in Cheetham Hill. That must be why they were called 'Red Recs' (Rec stands for recreation). The 'Red Rec' is often mentioned in TV programmes such as Coronation Street. I wonder if the programme-makers know where the name 'Red Rec' originated, because they are still using the name Red Rec even though the red brick shale has long gone and the fields are covered with grass now. Anyway, it saved the Corporation some money not having to pay for a groundsman to keep the grass mown and tidy; money was scarce in those austere days not long after the war.

We travelled everywhere by bus or train or walked. In those days very few people could afford motor cars. A few deaf people had motorbikes and some had bicycles, but with my balance problems I stuck to travelling by bus or train. I remember once we had played football against the Liverpool Deaf Club. We stayed to have a few pints with the Liverpool lads and one drink led to another, with the result that we missed the last train home. After talking about what was to be done, some could just about afford to stay in a bed and breakfast, but four of us didn't have enough money for that, so we decided that there was nothing else for it but to walk home. After finding the East Lancashire Road (A580) and getting our bearings, it was a straight walk of about 30 miles to home. Luckily it was a clear night, not a drop of rain, and with the moon and stars bright up above lighting our way and guiding us, we made our unsteady way home. The occasional shooting star flashing by overhead added to the enjoyment of such a magical night. We were young lads and so easily pleased in those days.

The sun was just coming up as we staggered into Salford; by then most of the enjoyment that we had started off with had evaporated. I had developed some massive blisters on my heels from that long walk and they were killing me. They were just about ready to pop when an early morning workman's bus came along. The bus driver stopped in response to our desperate waving, and with a sigh of relief we got on and sat down at last. Alighting in Piccadilly bus station we went our separate ways home. Luckily for me next day was Saturday and I didn't have to go to work, so I spent most of that Saturday in bed recovering and letting my blisters heal.

Fighting for our lives

In the battle of life it is not the critic who counts;
not the man who points out how the strong man
stumbled, or where the doer of a deed could have
done better. The credit belongs to the man who is
actually in the arena. Whose face is marred by dust
and sweat and blood; who strives valiantly; who
errs and comes short again and again, because
there is not effort without error and shortcoming;
who does actually strive to do the deeds; who
knows the great enthusiasms, the great devotions,
spends himself in a worthy cause; who at the best
knows at the end the triumph of high achievement;
and who at the worst, if he fails while daring
greatly, so that his place shall never be with those
cold and timid souls who have tasted neither
victory or defeat
Theodore Roosevelt

BEING DEAF CAN cause many misunderstandings
when trying to communicate with the hearing community,
sometimes with tragic results, but more often with hilarious
consequences, I suppose it all depends on your sense of
humour, which we deaf people really must keep if we wish
to remain sane. One story was related to me by a deaf friend
from Liverpool, where there are many natural comics. He
swears this truly happened to him and it is much funnier
when told by this Liverpool lad in sign language than I can
hope to do in writing, but I will try my best, so here goes.

One Saturday night our hero, let's call him Jim, had imbibed too much of the very tasty Liverpool beer at the Liverpool Deaf Club. Later that night, as Jim was wending his way home, he was staggering about on the pavement, partly from the amount of beer he had drunk and partly from his poor sense of balance as a result of being deaf. Jim thought he would take the easy way, so he flagged down a passing taxi which pulled into the kerb for him. Our Jim sat in the back seat, gave a sigh of relief and contentment and promptly fell asleep. Now this part of the story is conjecture because he was fast asleep and didn't know what was happening, but it was easy to guess. The taxi drove off and the driver spoke to our Jim asking him where he wanted to go. He of course was fast asleep, and also deaf, so he never answered the taxi driver, who repeated his request several times without getting an answer. The taxi driver must have thought, "Gosh! This man has had a heart attack, he must be dead," so he pulled over and phoned for an ambulance. Now back to the hero of the story.

Our hero, still in a daze, was suddenly awoken from his drunken slumber by medics easing him out of the taxi and strapping him onto a stretcher, pressing rhythmically on his chest and putting an oxygen mask on his face and getting their electrical apparatus ready to shock his heart back into action. As his arms were strapped down onto the stretcher and he had an oxygen mask on his face, he couldn't tell them that he was alright. Can you imagine the panic that ensued? He was imagining them sticking big needles into him and giving him electric shock treatment, so he started squirming and shaking his head and making blood-curdling, gurgling sounds. The medic commented: "Oh, good, he's back with us. Don't worry lad," he continued as he patted Jim on the head, "Stay with us and you'll be ok." They took him to the hospital and kept him in all night for observation, despite him insisting that he was alright and had only fallen asleep. They couldn't understand what he was trying to tell them and so they were taking no chances. He was able to explain what had happened the next day and so was allowed to go home.

In my opinion Deaf people are far and away much more interesting people and much more inventive than their hearing counterparts, who to me at least, seem to have such dull and boring lives compared to my deaf friends, but then I'm very biased. I hope that these statements have woken up a few dead brain cells and made people really think about what it means to be Deaf. It really is very hard for deaf people to try to get on in the hearing world but; EXCUSES ARE FOR LOSERS. Winners meet life's challenges head on knowing that there are no guarantees, and give it all they have got, so come on you deafies, be more assertive. It's never too late or too early to begin to take control of your life. Time plays no favourites and will pass whether you act or not. Dare to dream and take risks, compete. If you are not willing to work for your goals, don't expect others to do it for you. BELIEVE IN YOURSELF.!

That last line is crucial. You must have confidence in yourself and what you are doing as you don't always have to look to hearing people for approval. Do it for yourself, nobody else. Becoming deaf is not such a great tragedy that it at first seemed to be, and if I had not become deaf, then I would never have met Diana, who has enriched my life so much.

Diana lived on the other side of Manchester, in Withington, which in those days was a posh part of Manchester, about 14 miles from Middleton where I lived, so in order to spend more time with her I packed in the football, and went direct from my job as a cutter for ladies mantles and costumes to Diana's home to take her out to the pictures or the deaf club on Grosvenor Street in Manchester. This deaf club had the legend, 'The Manchester Institute for the Deaf' carved in stone over the front entrance. It was a very popular place for Deaf people to gather and meet other deaf people. Many outings, sports, hobbies, dances etc were organised there. I used to love going with some of them out into the Derbyshire countryside and rambling all over the Peak District and filling my lungs with the fresh clean air, which after working all week in the clothing factory was badly needed.

This place on Grosvenor Street was very popular and it had served the deaf community for over 100 years, so it was a shock to many deaf people when it was closed some time in the 1970s and we were given a place on Booth Street East not far away. We were told that the university owned the land and wanted it back for some building they were planning, but the old building on Grosvenor Street is still there to this day over 30 years after we were evicted. It is now a very popular and profitable night club called 'The Deaf Institute'. Incidentally, when going there on the bus in those bygone days, I would pronounced it 'Gros-ven-or Street' and had some strange looks from bus conductors when I asked for a ticket to 'Gros-ven-or Street'. They didn't seem to know where Gros-venor- Street was. When I explained to my sister Patricia, she corrected me. "It's 'Gro-ve-nor, with a silent 'S'," she said. I still had a long way to go until my pronunciation was correct. Patricia had instilled in me a love of books and reading, and so while my love of reading had helped me tremendously in improving my use of the English language, it did not help me to pronounce many words correctly. It was necessary to be able to hear to enable a person to copy the right way to say a word.

I would advise any deaf person who wants to improve his/her English to read books, magazines, newspapers etc, and especially read something that you are interested in about your hobbies or work, note the order in which the words are arranged, read something every day, read more some days than others, take your time and read the words thoroughly, try to follow the context, try to understand what the words mean, and have a dictionary at hand for when you come across a difficult word. Remember that many books are printed that don't deserve to be, so don't believe everything that you read. This practice is to help you to understand the English language. Try to relate one book to another and all the books you read to life in general and your own experiences, it is only by reading in this manner that the most joy and value is to be obtained from books. You may have gathered from all this that I am rather fond of books and reading. I have my sister Patricia to thank for that, and I believe that the more you read the better your English becomes.

Ever since I was a kid I have loved books. Everything about a real book evokes memories of the happiest times of my life. Books bring back memories of the love and closeness I felt for my sister Patricia. I love the feel, sight and smell of books, old and new. Books were always a refuge for me and a ticket to dreamland. They allowed me to travel the world without leaving my bedroom. Books allowed me, for a brief time, to forget my deafness, I could in my imagination hold conversations with many famous people, dead or alive. Yes; books are a delight. Growing up in a time before subtitles on both films and television, books were for me a gateway into the wide world.

I would also see Diana every Sunday at Father Hayward's church/club at 431 Chester Road. Some of the other deaf people would travel long distances to attend Mass there. They came from as far as Liverpool, Preston, Rochdale and other far-flung places. They would write down their weekly confessions on slips of paper and there would be much giggling between Diana, Pat, Winnie, Moira and the other girls as they were writing their confessions with their heads close together. It made me wonder what sort of sins they were confessing. Or were they just pleased to see each other again.

After confession we went to Mass, which the priest said in Latin with his back to us. This was a pity because I would have loved to see him signing in Latin, if it was possible. Then we received our weekly Holy Communion. Incidentally, a young lad well known in the Deaf world named Terry Riley was the altar boy at these masses. Most of us would bring sandwiches and brew tea after Mass and spend the day in signed conversation. For many it must have been a relief and very relaxing to have someone to converse with after spending all week in isolation in the hearing world.

This priest ruled his little world with an iron fist. He would give advice on a variety of subjects, including marriage problems, which made me think what did he, a single man know about sex and marriage? How on earth could he give advice on sexual problems when the very word 'Sex' was taboo? Or did he have a secret life? He gave advice on all aspects of daily living, even gaving advice on such personal topics as which person it was suitable to marry, and who should and who shouldn't marry. In the 1950s hypocrisy was still thriving as much as it was in Victorian times. He persuaded some of the members to form a teetotal club and wear badges and try to recruit as many members as possible, and to proclaim proudly to the world that they never touched a drop of alcohol, which he said was evil as well as bad for your health (Jesus drank wine), but he then said that smoking was alright (Jesus didn't smoke but he himself smoked like a chimney, both cigarettes and a pipe). This is another fine example of the wrong person in a position of authority giving bad advice. His teeth were stained yellow from the nicotine, he smoked a brand of tobacco called Three Nuns. I suppose it was a quick way to get to Heaven. He was definitely not my kind of man. I like to keep a bit of distance between myself and any person who insists that his way is the only way to go. Needless to say, I didn't join his teetotal club, the very thought was enough to send shivers of dread running up and down my spine. It must be the Irish in me. My Mam even put some Guinness into the stews that she made for us. I couldn't imagine eating it without some Guinness in it.

In those simple, innocent days of the 1950s, pre-mobile phones, subtitles on TV (never mind pre-subtitles, many of us didn't even have a TV until sometime in the late 1960s), pre-DVD's, health and safety, human rights, pre-steroids for sports, pre-equal opportunities, race relations, etc, etc, the priest would organise Christmas parties to be held in an upstairs room in the public library on Stretford Road. The girls were told not to wear high heels as they would mark the parquet floor. Diana did not like that at all as she was very fond of her killer heels. As you can imagine, there were no alcoholic drinks, just lashings of cups of tea poured from a big enamel tea pot. The tea was made from the boiling water drawn from a huge gas-fired stainless steel urn that rattled and shook and emitted gusts of steam as it boiled, reminiscent of the boiler on a steamroller. There were also sausage rolls, spam or cheese sandwiches and cakes.

This era was before Bill Haley and his Comets burst upon the scene with 'Rock around the Clock' and sent the youth of the time into a wild frenzy and gave birth to Teddy boys and Teddy girls, so the dances were very discreet waltzes and quicksteps, with maybe a Gay Gordon thrown in if you felt brave enough to defy the priest's disapproving glare. You had to hold your girl respectfully, with a visible distance between both of you. The priest would sit in a chair leaning forward with his chin resting on his hands that were folded on top of his walking stick held between his knees, with his eagle eye scanning the dancers to make sure that no hanky panky was going on. Strangely enough all enjoyed themselves. When the music ended, the deaf people would carry on dancing, so a man would go round tapping them on the shoulder and telling them to stop dancing as the music had finished. Meantime the pub around the corner, the Cumberland Hotel, would be packed with deaf people who had heard that a party was going on, but preferred to have a few drinks in the nearby pub and meet old friends there away from the priest's steely gaze. Friendships formed in the deaf institutions would very often last for life and deaf people would travel miles to meet their old friends. One of the lads told me that the pub was packed with deaf people from far and wide, The famous Pink brothers, Stephen and Tony, had come from far away London. I told Diana and she said, "Let's go and see", so we slipped out unnoticed and went to see them. We had a very enjoyable time talking about the old days at Boston Spa.

One of the most popular deaf couples in the Manchester deaf scene of those days in the 1950/60s were Mr. Terry Riley and his wife Mary, the parents of the present British Deaf Association Honorary Chairman, also called Terry Riley, who along with his younger brother Kevin were little boys at that time. Their sister Maria would not be born until a few years later. Their home was like another 'Deaf Club'. Any deaf people who had enjoyed themselves so much and had taken such a long time to say a reluctant goodbye that they had missed the last bus or train home were always welcome to spend the night at their home. Oh yes! They were good days, I have many fond memories of those days and they shall remain fond memories. As well as all those good things, I think that I should mention that beer came in oak barrels, not metal casks, and the taste was far superior, so you see progress is not always for the better.

Most Sundays we would usually start saying our goodbyes at about 1pm, and making our way home, as Fr Hayward was by that time in need of his afternoon nap. I would take Diana to her home in Withington, then spend the rest of the day there with her and her parents. Diana's mum always invited me to have dinner with them. I never refused as she was an excellent cook and she would often cook some really exotic dishes. Her chicken curry was out of this world, and Diana has inherited her mum's skill in the kitchen. My mam was a good cook too, but her cooking was good old plain English food, her ham hock and pea soup was very tasty, so I was well fed and beginning to put some serious muscle on from my active life. After spending an enjoyable evening with Diana I would get the bus from Withington into town and from there get another bus to Victoria Avenue in Blackley, and from there I would walk the remaining three miles home because in those days there were no buses to Middleton from Manchester after 11pm and very few people could afford taxis.

One very cold winter's night, well past midnight, as I was wending my way home from an enjoyable evening at Diana's house, I was walking along Manchester New Road. It had been snowing heavily the past week and the snow had been shovelled into heaps along the kerb of the road. As I was walking along, my mind was dwelling on the lovely evening that I had just spent with Diana and my head was up in the clouds, so I never noticed the four soldiers until I was right on top of them. I know I should have stepped into the snow and let them pass, but I wasn't thinking right, I said, "Excuse me, lads" and just sidled my way through them. As I passed through, one of them turned and kicked me on my bum. I should have carried on walking or even burst into a run, but being me, the silly fool that I am, I turned on them and said, "What did you do that for?" They grabbed me and pushed me up against a wall. I could smell the alcohol on their breath. They said something to me, I said "I'm sorry, I can't hear you" and then I craned my head forward to try to catch what they were saying. That's when the fist caught me right on my nose. I was unprepared for it, I didn't see it coming, and the blow sent tears into my eyes and stars exploding around me and I went down.

At that time of night there was nobody about, so they took their time booting me all over the road. After a time three of them stopped, but the fourth carried on kicking me. He was in frenzy and I think the others were trying to stop him, but he seemed to be going berserk. After kicking me some more he grabbed hold of one of my legs and dragged me into the middle of the road. He had stopped kicking while he was dragging me and this gave me a chance to clear my head. He must have thought there was no fight in me because I had not hit back or attempted to defend myself as I was unprepared for their attack on me and in a state of shock. He then stood astride me and reached down to grab my coat. That's when I exploded with my left foot smack into his testicles, or as we say in Collyhurst "his bollocks". While he was rolling about on the road screaming in agony, I rolled over and got to my feet. His mates made a half-hearted move towards me. I wiped the blood away from my eyes and looked at them. This time I was ready for another onslaught, but there must have been something in the look I gave them, or they must have felt bad about what they had done, because they left me alone. They turned to help their mate, who was squirming and moaning in pain on the road, and I turned and stumbled along the road towards home.

My eyes were narrow slits through the swelling and I could barely see as I staggered along the road making my painful way home. I have been reliably informed that in the army only officers have 'testicles'. NCOs have 'balls' and privates have common or garden 'bollocks'. Whatever you want to call them, a well-aimed kick in that vulnerable place will bring the biggest man down. And that brings to mind those immortal words from 'Colonel Bogy':

Hitler has only got one ball.
Goering has two, but very small

32

Himmler has something similar
But poor old Goebbels has no balls at all

So from that information I deduced that they must have been privates.

Next morning I had two black eyes, a swollen nose and I was covered in bruises. I felt as if I had some broken ribs, but luckily as it later transpired it was a false alarm. I was spitting fire and swearing vengeance. My poor mam was shocked at my appearance. I think she was beginning to think that she had a hooligan for a son living in her house. I had to explain to my brother Jimmy what had happened. He said, "There's a Territorial Army place just at the bottom of Manchester New Road, they must have come from there." Jimmy went to see some of his old Collyhurst mates and together we waited outside the army depot for several nights. There were six of us, Jimmy and me and four of Jimmy's mates from Collyhurst. Every time a soldier walked past they would ask me, "Is that one of 'em Kev?" No! This carried on for a few nights with no sign of the soldiers who had attacked me. I was beginning to forget what they looked like. Then one night I caught a glimpse of one of them. I pointed him out to Jimmy and we waited for the others to appear. After a few nights of non-appearance I gave up waiting for those soldiers, that blazing anger and thirst for vengeance had faded with the passage of time and I had better things to do, like courting Diana. But Jimmy and his mates must have carried on waiting for them because one day Jimmy said to me, "Kev. They won't bother you again." By then I had lost interest, so I didn't ask him what had happened.

I had eased up on my training and was just messing about doing body weight exercises from the old Charles Atlas course when I felt like it. But this incident made me determined to become hard and strong again using heavy weights and punch bag, so I went back to 'Mr. Manchester' Ken Latham's weightlifting club. I had let my membership lapse when I met Diana, so I signed on again and began training in a frenzy. Ken had to tell me to calm down, to take it slowly. I told him what had happened and I was determined that nobody was ever going to beat me up again, and to this day nobody ever has. What must be understood about Ken Latham's weight lifting club is that unlike modern day, so-called gyms, with their polished floors and potted ferns, where you are not allowed to use heavy weights in case you rupture yourself or damage the floor, Ken's gym was just an old double garage in his mother-in-laws garden. It consisted of lots of heavy weights, both barbells and dumbbells, benches, abdominal boards etc., nothing fancy but enough hard core equipment to frighten off the ones who were not serious about their training. The most valuable thing, that I am unable to put a price tag on, was Ken's knowledge of how to build muscle and get freaky strong, as it was known in the pre-steroid days. We never became heavyweight monsters like today's weightlifters, but we were certainly stronger.

In the 1950s I was a subscriber to the old British magazine called Health and Strength. I picked up lots of useful information from it. Once there was an article about a world champion weightlifter named Doug Hepburn. He was giving an interview and answering a lot of questions. He had come to England on his way back to Canada from a weightlifting competition somewhere in Europe. I missed meeting him, but from his photos he looked as big as a brick outhouse, apart from his right leg which had been puny and shrivelled from birth. From the way he answered the questions, I could see that he was a very sensitive man, but he also gave a lot of valuable advice. Despite being born with a club foot he became the heavyweight champion weightlifter of the world and Olympic gold medalist. He was also born with a very bad squint in his eyes, which was corrected by surgery in infancy, so he certainly wasn't born with good genetics. How can you not admire such will power? This is a poem that he composed.

> *I know I'm not wrong*
> *And the struggle is clean*
> *I'll keep pushing on*
> *And I'll never turn mean*
> *There aren't very many*
> *Who can see how I've tried*
> *There's a lot think they know*
> *But not deep down inside*
> *You're certain to win*
> *If you push right on through*
> *And if you never give in*
> *Your dream will come true.*

I think that is a fitting poem for many deaf people who have had to struggle a lot in their lives too, that's why I'm including it in my story.

The Language of Deafness

Great spirits have always found violent
opposition from mediocrities
Albert Einstein

IN THE GOOD old days, or bad old days depending on which side you were looking at it from, before the hearing world realised that money could be made from sign language, signing was despised by them (The Hearing People). It was looked upon as an inferior method of communication. There was also a stigma attached to being deaf on a par with those people who had mental illness. Deaf people suffered terrible discrimination from hearing people, which even made many deaf people ashamed to be seen signing in public. They would always try to sign inconspicuously, with many a furtive glance around to make sure that nobody was watching them, and thus their own language had become something to be ashamed of. I know of some deaf people who as kids were put in the cupboard under the stairs whenever the family had visitors, just like in 'Harry Potter'. It seems hard to believe nowadays that some deaf people were even placed in mental asylums, with their only problem being that they couldn't communicate with hearing people. There was nothing wrong with their brains! The problem of being deaf, though it's bad enough, is not the worst problem; far worse is the attitude of many hearing people towards the deaf.

Many hearing people consider deaf people to be simple-minded and treat them as such. Many deaf people have never been taught the English language, so you can see that it's not surprising at all why so many deaf people developed massive inferiority complexes. I am convinced that this is the reason why there are so many deaf people who, understandably, try to build up their self-esteem by making up fantastic stories about themselves; many have developed real 'Walter Mitty' personalities.

Then some hearing people started sign language classes. They recruited some deaf people to be the tutors, and to fully exploit the situation they decided to use the old Roman ploy of divide and rule. Suddenly, where we had only sign language before, we now had BSL, SSE, and makaton, whatever that is! Then there was 'cued speech', though I had never seen any deaf people using this method, and some other variations of sign language. What had once been a beautiful expressive language had become complicated; unity had been replaced by separate schools of thought, each of which snubbed the other. If someone tells you that their method of signing is best, run away quickly, especially if they are hearing people who don't have a clue about what it is like to be deaf, but think they do, like UFOs, Bigfoot, Yetis and the lost city of Atlantis, to really understand the deaf you must have hearing problems yourself.

Deaf people are a strange and mysterious topic to many hearing people, and many of those who do get to know deaf people and learn how to communicate with them seem to think that we are a simple-minded people and need them to tell us what to do. One good thing to come from this is all these sign language classes have made many more hearing people 'deaf-aware'.

Throughout history deafness has been widely misunderstood, with deaf people labelled as 'stupid', 'idiotic', 'bad tempered' or 'dangerous'. It's so frustrating and many deaf lads cannot handle it. If a deaf man starts a fight in a pub then all deaf people are barred from that pub. If a hearing man starts a fight in the pub then only that man is barred from that pub. The reasoning behind it is that deaf people are all the same, they are all placed in the same box. But is not so with hearing people, who are all individuals and must be treated as such. It is attitudes like this that make deaf people feel they are inferior and second class citizens.

In my humble opinion as a deaf man who would do anything for a peaceful life, I believe in my old Irish granny's favourite saying, 'Live and Let Live', and I try to live by that rule. I have always tried not to force my opinions on other people, but when I read about hearing people who don't have a clue what is involved in being deaf, sprouting a lot of nonsense, then I must say that I think that deaf people's sign language should have been left alone by hearing 'experts'. Deaf people didn't divide their language into separate signing methods, BSL in one corner, SSE in the other, and handbags at dawn. We didn't engage in silly arguments about which was the best or worse, and we certainly didn't close our minds to the method of signing that would help us best to gain more knowledge (Total Communication). We were told that the sign language that deaf people had used for hundreds of years was all wrong and that we must change and sign their way.

When I was a little kid before I became deaf, I can remember that my mum was fond of singing 'Galway Bay', amongst other songs, as she went about her daily chores, scrubbing out the scullery or donkey-stoning the front step. Years later, when remembering back with a certain amount of nostalgia, I could still hear the music of that song in my mind's ear (why not?). It had a haunting melody that kept going over and over in my mind. So I decided to find the lyrics of that song, and after some searching on my computer I found the words and so I was able to put the lyrics to the music. Some of the words struck me as being very evocative of the problems that deaf people, and the Gaelic people, were having with other people trying to interfere with their language. I thought those words were very apt for the situation that deaf people find themselves in today:

The strangers came and tried to teach us their ways
They scorned us just for being what we are
But they might as well try chasing after moonbeams
Or light a penny candle from a star

I can remember in the old days there were many deaf people who were brilliant signers and so erudite they always had an audience who were mesmerised by their skilled, expressive signing. My old scoutmaster, Mr Caproni from Boston Spa was one such person. His adventure stories and tales of derring do, especially his stories about two cowboys named 'Deaf Smith' and 'Jim Hatfield', who were the scourge of all the baddies in the Wild West. His stories used to keep us kids enthralled every Wednesday and Friday evening at St John's. He didn't just tell the stories he became Deaf Smith or D'Artagnan or Athos, or whoever the story was about. It was sheer magic to watch.

Other deaf people were not such good signers. Just as there are great and poor speakers in the hearing world, there are great and poor signers in the deaf world. In the hearing world great speakers are said to have the gift of the gab. That gift could be used for good or bad. Winston Churchill used his oratory skills to rally the British people and the Empire to defeat Adolf Hitler. Hitler was another great orator, but he used his speaking skills for evil. Somehow Adolf Hitler cast a spell over the German people with his oratory skills and convinced them that Jews, gypsies, those with mental illnesses, deaf people and other so-called undesirables had to be eliminated. In Germany sterilisations of deaf, mentally ill and other disabled people began in 1934 and continued all through the war, resulting in estimates of 300,000 to 400,000 sterilisations. The Nazis targeted mental hospitals, deaf institutions and care homes. During the war they went on to exterminate approximately 200,000 to 250,000 people who were considered mentally or physically disabled.

Since those dreadful times studies from the 1950s into public attitudes to deafness has revealed how deafness has been stigmatized throughout history. St Augustine, an early Christian saint, stated that deaf people cannot go to Heaven; to gain entry into Heaven you must be able to hear the word of God. Now fancy that! I'd better start praying harder! You may think that I'm exaggerating and being very cynical, but I'm not. That's the way it was. Luckily most grassroots deaf people turned a deaf ear (whoops!) to those busybodies trying to tell them how to sign. Sign language evolves naturally and is not static. It doesn't stagnate, new words and things are continually being invented and they need a new sign for them, and deaf people are quite capable of doing that for themselves. One thing that all deaf people have in common when signing, the thing that sets them apart from hearing people who can sign, is a very expressive body language and facial expressions.

There were many deaf people who thought it was wrong that hearing people should have such strong views on how deaf people should sign, but the opinions of those deaf people were just ignored. My observations of human nature have left me somewhat, shall I say, 'underwhelmed'. There are few people in the deaf world that have any visibility, who speak on behalf of the true interests of typical grassroots deaf people. Most deaf people with visibility speak on behalf of the hearing establishment and therefore have to peddle the 'company line'. When they were recruiting deaf people to be tutors of sign language they selected the ones who they thought were easy to manipulate and do what they were told, not the ones who had minds of their own.

Those deaf people, including myself, who showed any signs of intelligence and literacy were rejected. Oh, no! Where money is involved they couldn't take the risk of having any deaf person with some intelligence seeing them for what they really were.

Those deaf people who were selected to be tutors even had to learn how to sign again. The fact that they had been signing all their lives made no difference; they had to pass stages 1, 2, 3 and 4, and pay over £1000 for a certificate to prove that they could sign. When I asked why the hearing people who were making money out of this scheme didn't have certificates to prove that they could speak, I was told that it wasn't necessary for them as they were all experts in the English language. So much for BSL. It seems that in those hearing people's eyes, those deaf people chosen to be tutors were not expert signers in their own language and needed to be taught how to sign properly, and had to pay for that privilege. Then the deaf people were split up into two different groups and put into different boxes: those born deaf were higher case D-Deaf people, while those who became deaf after having been born hearing were lower case d-deaf people. Doing things like this is always a dangerous practice. Many people thought that it insinuated that those described with a capital D were somehow superior to those who were merely described as lower case d. In 1930s Germany a certain Josef Goebbels was an expert at categorising people into superior and inferior sects, and we people of a certain age know where that practice led to, don't we?

As well as hearing people, many deaf people are not going to like that analysis. Nonetheless it is the simple truth as I see it. I have no axe to grind at my age, I am just stating the truth as I see it and from talking to other deaf people and sometimes when the truth hurts, only a lie appears to be beautiful. Where are those deaf sign language tutors now?

The hearing people who recruited them began sending them letters and pamphlets explaining rule changes and meetings etc in legalised English using very big words. BSL has no written language, and as they were BSL users and BSL was their only method of communication they had no knowledge of English grammar. They couldn't understand the letters being sent to them and became so frustrated and disheartened that they pulled out of tutoring sign language. They were trying to teach BSL sign language and its 'unique grammar' to hearing people, while at the same time trying to make sense of the correspondence involved in teaching that was written in perfect English. They just couldn't understand it. It was too stressful for them. The deaf people who stuck to the tutoring were the ones with a good grasp of the English language.

I think that we have a contradiction in terms here. You must be good at the English language to be able to teach BSL, which doesn't use English grammar. In fact, BSL doesn't have a written language at all. Everything that we know about ourselves comes from recorded history. Even the cavemen tried to keep records with their paintings on the walls of caves. The main difference separating the human race from animals is our ability to read and write. Humans have a written language, we record our lives and it is from these records that we have learned and progressed. Reading those records allows us to look back at the past with objectivity. We can analyse the past and see where we went either right or wrong. This allows us to learn from the past and with that knowledge we can shape the future. That is why I consider SSE to be so important for deaf children to learn. O what a tangled web we weave! If you can understand why some people think that BSL is so much more important, will you please explain it to me, because surely signing following the written and spoken word is the logical way to go.

Becoming deaf had opened up a whole new world for me. I had deaf friends all over Britain from my days at St John's. I had friends in London, Liverpool, Leeds, Blackpool, Carlisle, Birmingham, in fact it seemed like I had friends and acquaintances in every town and city in Britain, and from the three Manchester deaf clubs I made many more brilliant friends.

Remembering St John's

*A morsel of genuine history is a thing so rare
as to be always valuable*
Thomas Jefferson - third President of the United States.

OVER 60 YEARS after leaving St John's, Boston Spa, here I am sitting in the doorway of my poly tunnel on my allotment breathing in the cool evening air. I have about 200 square metres of very fertile land that has received an annual load of horse manure for the past 30 years. It's a 10ft x 25ft poly tunnel in which I grow tomatoes, cucumbers, peppers, chillies etc. I am sitting on an old rickety plastic chair that is threatening to collapse under me, with my feet propped up on a bag of potting compost. I have just poured myself a cup of tea from my thermos flask and I'm giving my back a much needed rest from the winter digging and manuring. As I sit there sipping tea, I am contemplating the meaning of life, trying to work out the secret of what makes a man irresistible to women and watching the leaves on the surrounding trees turning to beautiful Autumn colours, gold, orange and various shades of brown and beginning to fall. I think the Americans have a very apt word for autumn; they call it the 'Fall', which sounds so much nicer. The sheer beauty of it all is enough to make me hold my breath and forget the discomfort from my damp socks and the water that had seeped through the hole in my welly. So you see there is some poetry in my soul, I am not all about being a macho he-man. I can be very sensitive, in fact I think that I would make a good counsellor. If I sit quietly I will sometimes see a stoat slinking through the bushes looking for a mouse for its dinner. Getting an allotment was one of the best things I ever did; I find it so relaxing. If only some people would leave me alone to enjoy it.

I think to myself, "Kev! It's 2011 and you are 76 years old (at the time of writing). Your kids are grown up, you have grandchildren taller than you now and your great grandchildren will soon be taller than you too (they already are, they call me a little munchkin). Where did all the years go? As my mind begins to wander back into the mists of those long gone days of my childhood, when the world had gone mad with countries trying to annihilate each other in 1940s wartime Britain, faces begin to appear there, long gone faces of my dead pals from St John's, Boston Spa. Mr. Caproni, Mr. Young (Foo Foo) and the lads, Billy Jones, Cyril Clarke, Willie Kelly, John Wilson, the two Adamus brothers from Poland, Brian Kelly, Danny Moynihan. I have never had such close friends in the hearing world as these lads. We were living close to each other, sharing the same experiences, playing together every day, sleeping in the same dormitory, helping each other. We forged bonds that were impossible to break, and often these friendships lasted for life. Many of these lads died long before their allotted three score and ten. Why was that? I have a theory. I think it has something to do with the rubbish food we were given in our formative years, partly due to the wartime shortage of food and also partly due to the fact that we were not given our full rations. And due to the difficulty that deaf people had in getting access to information from their doctors, and the communication problems they have when they finally do manage to get access to their doctors. These lads had very poor English because of the idiotic education methods in use for deaf children at that time. They couldn't read and write as good as their hearing counterparts, nor ccould they hear or talk, so they didn't enjoy the same access to the information from the NHS that hearing people had. They were treated as if they were defective human beings who were second class people. If they didn't develop that strong sense of scepticism and inner strength to enable them to survive the slings and arrows that life would throw at them, then they were on the slippery downward spiral into mental problems, alcoholism and an early death that was the fate of many of my deaf school friends. Many of them were not prepared for the life outside the Institution; it was a big shock to realise that they couldn't speak as well as they had been led to believe they could.

Now why have these faces come back to haunt me? Is it because it is All Souls' Day, or as our American friends call it 'Halloween', a time when long gone souls are roaming the world trying to find peace. As I sat there on that rickety plastic chair I was feeling melancholy as deep in reverie I let my mind drift back to those long gone days at St John's Institution for the Deaf and Dumb. Those long dead deaf friends of mine certainly didn't find peace here in this world, did they? Or are they trying to tell me something? Were the Sisters right and they are trying to tell me that they are in Heaven? Or Is Billy Jones trying to tell me that he is in Hell because he fell in love with and married a proddy girl? After all, the Sisters had told us often enough that we must marry a good Catholic girl, and have lots of good Catholic children, as if God would be bothered about a little detail like was a person a Catholic or a Protestant. The important thing is that you are a good person and live your life without hurting anyone else, then God will be pleased with you, never mind what your religious beliefs are. Or what about Danny? Is he in Hell too because he drank too much? Surely God will understand that he drank to blot out the pain and stress of trying to live in a world that is not designed for deaf people. What about Val? Is he in Hell because he was always telling fibs and forgot to confess it? He was only doing that because he lacked confidence in himself. No! I don't think God could be angry with these lads, they went straight to Heaven, of that I am sure. They already had their Hell here on Earth when they were alive and trying to live in a hearing world that is not designed for deaf people.

In my humble opinion, for what it's worth, deafness is a far worse affliction than blindness. Ss the deaf/blind lady Helen Keller once said, "Deafness cuts you off from people, blindness merely cuts you off from things." She also said, "The best and most beautiful things in the world cannot be seen or even touched, they must be felt with the heart." What a great lady she must have been. I would love to have met her. She must have been an exceptionally intelligent lady, as the way she coped with such a terrible affliction was amazing. Being deaf is bad enough, but to be both deaf and blind, I can't imagine what that must be like. At the recent Boston Spa reunion there was a young girl who was deaf/blind and was accompanied by a lady minder. At breakfast in the hotel the morning after the reunion party I noticed this young girl trying to explain through finger spelling that she wanted flora with her toast. Her minder couldn't seem to understand what she was saying. I watched her signing 'flora' a few times and the minder looking puzzled, so I stepped in and told the minder that the girl wanted flora. The minder looked relieved and thanked me, but it made me wonder what kind of qualifications she had to be in charge of such a vulnerable young girl.

Come on Kev, push these morbid thoughts out of your mind. Do you mean to tell me that after all these years your experiences at St John's still affect you? Well, some things that happened there are very hard to forget. For instance, I have difficulty forgetting the dental surgery in the corridor opposite the classrooms. It still makes me shudder when I think of it. I have a problem forgetting the pedal-operated drill the dentist used on us, and also I have a problem in that

I cannot remember the dentist ever using any anaesthetics, but I can remember the excruciating pain when the drill touched a nerve, and I can remember vividly the queue of little boys waiting their turn outside that dreaded room, all of them trembling with fear and wanting their mam, and the occasional scream coming from behind that door that even I could hear. I remember how the dentist, his face flushed and angry, would tell Sister Margaret to make us behave and to stop struggling and she would angrily berate us for letting the school down with our snivelling. There were no lollipops for us little brats. I have been told that abuse and bullying like that was happening in hearing schools to kids too. The difference was, those hearing kids could go home after school and be back with their families. That was denied to us - we might just as well have been prisoners.

I can still remember the bitter cold winter of 1946-47. The biting cold really began in autumn of 1946 and lasted to the spring of 1947. In January of 1947 it began to get really cold, it snowed for days on end. The whole country came to a standstill, trains and buses stopped running, the roads were impassable, many old people froze to death in the intense cold. It was like we were in another ice age, the cold was everywhere, there was no escaping it. When the wind blew the chill factor made it feel even colder, even in bed two blankets were not enough. My last thought before I went to sleep was, "Brrr! It's c-c-c-old". During the day we wore a vest and a jersey, corduroy jerkins, short corduroy trousers and stockings and boots. Most of the time our feet were like blocks of ice, our legs were pink from the cold, our faces were like beetroots. Many of the lads suffered from chilblains and the skin between their fingers was cracked and raw. Sister Mary, who was in charge of the clinic, would put a greasy ointment on their hands and it burnt as it went into the cracks. I remember clearly seeing the label. It was called 'Snowfire'. Playing football was impossible, the snow on the football field had been impacted into a solid sheet of ice about 12 inches thick, a mini ice age indeed. And so, instead of football we invented a game to be played in the shed that was situated at the top end of the playground. It was quite a large shed with one side open to the playground, about 50 to 60 feet long. We used a small ball like a tennis ball and the rules were the ball must not touch the ground, no using hands, you must first kick the ball up to hit the roof then try to get a goal as it came down while not letting the ball touch the ground. We quickly became very adept and nimble-footed at keeping the ball off the ground and bouncing the ball off the wall, then running round your opponent to catch it on the rebound on the other side of him before it hit the ground. We would soon work up a sweat despite the bitter cold and our breath came in clouds of steam, but we couldn't keep it up for long because other kids were standing about shivering awaiting their turns, so the rules were altered to allow five lads a side to play. So I wonder if five-a-side football originated at St John's, Boston Spa in the 1940s?

When I went home for the holidays I was able to run rings round the hearing lads when we played football against the lads from other streets, thanks to the game we played in the shed at St John's. There were a lot of lads who became good footballers who picked up their ball control skills by playing in the streets of northern towns – Francis Lee, Brian Kidd, Mike Summerbee, Tom Finney, Stan Mathews, David Pegg, Paul Scholes, Nobby Stiles and many more who all began playing football in the 'Back Street League' long before they became professionals. Nowadays little kids go to these 'football academies' to learn how to play the game. Is that why there are so few individuals in the game now? I am sure there were many deaf lads who were just as good, if not better, footballers than those who I have just mentioned, but because of communication difficulties these deaf lads were not given the same opportunities as the hearing lads. But I am digressing, so back to St John's.

At St Johns we turned the playground into an ice skating rink. At night before we went to bed we would empty buckets of water all over the playground, gangs of little lads would be seen carrying buckets of water from the wash room and being directed where to empty them by some bigger boys. In the bitter cold it wouldn't take long for this water to freeze solid and make a great ice skating rink. Next morning after Mass and breakfast, and for a few minutes before school, we tried it out. Previously we had been to the cobblers shop to knock some metal studs into our boot soles because we could skate better with them. Metal on ice was much better that leather on ice, so you see, we did try to turn that bitter winter to our advantage and have a bit of fun.

In the scout hut there was a rusty cast iron pot-bellied stove in one corner which we had never seen being used before. I suggested to Cyril, Willie Kelly and Billy Jones that we should clean it up, gather some wood and light a fire in it and get warm. We all agreed that it was a good idea, so we got a stockpile of scrap wood from the wood shed and joiner's shop. The next problem to solve was how to light it as we had no matches. We sat down and discussed ways and means. Various methods involving magnifying glasses and rubbing sticks together were suggested and discarded as there was no sun for the magnifying glass and rubbing sticks together seemed too daft. Willie came up with the best idea. He said that he could go down to the boiler room when the caretaker had gone for his dinner and get some hot coals from the boiler, but what to carry hot coals in? Also, he had to be fast before the coals lost their heat in the bitter cold. A metal container was found and Willie set off to get the hot coals whilst I went to the toilets to get some of the squares of newspaper that were used for wiping our bums. Willie came running back with the coals and put them in the stove, then I piled the newspaper on and some sticks. Nothing happened at first, but luckily from my experiences of my Collyhurst days I knew what to do. I bent down and blew on the coals and paper until it ignited, then more paper and sticks, and soon it was blazing merrily away. We also purloined some coal from the boiler house, the warmth felt lovely, we had left the little door open so that we could feel the warmth better.

You could really feel the cold if you moved away from the stove, so there was some competition for the best positions, pushing, pulling and jostling, trying to hold our ground. Billy Jones, being the biggest lad, had pushed his way to the front. We stood there in front of the open stove door, embracing the lovely warmth, although our fronts were lovely and warm our backs were still very cold. We found it best to turn round slowly so that we were well done on both sides. Then Billy noticed that because he was standing so close to the fire, he was getting mottled red lines on his legs where they were burning, so we all moved back but didn't leave the warmth of the scout shed until dinner time. We did that all through that bitter winter until the cold weather eased up at Easter. Mr. Harker, the joinery instructor, must have wondered where all the off cuts of wood had gone. Some of the fencing had gone too. In order to keep our secret of keeping warm in the bitter cold we had to promise not to tell anybody else, only the 15-16 year olds. But I suspected that Mr Caproni knew because I would sometimes catch him looking at some of us and chuckling quietly to himself. He was probably giving us points for using our initiative.

What has been will be again, what has been done will be done again;
there is nothing new under the sun
Ecclesiastes

At one of the annual Boston Spa reunions some of the women told me that it was the same on the girl's side too. The Sisters made their lives miserable with the constant praying and lecturing against evil, especially evil boys, whom they must not look at. Once some of the senior girls rebelled against such oppression. They thought that surely this is not the way God intended them to live, surely this is not what Jesus meant when he said, "Suffer Little Children to come to Me". If God loved them and was kind like the Sisters say, then why were they told that they would go to Hell and suffer for eternity just for looking at boys. Was God wrong to make boys? It just didn't make sense. Four of the senior girls decided that they had had enough and they were so unhappy that they would run away. It was really a cry for help, and they hoped that by running away they would draw attention to what was happening to them at St John's. I won't say any names as they may not want people to know about it after all these years, they may not even be alive now. They were eventually caught by the police and brought back to the Institution, and from what I was told they were very badly treated by the Sisters. They were man-handled, smacked, had their hair pulled, shouted at and pushed about, and threatened with Hellfire and damnation for evermore, until, that is, one of the girls snapped. She grabbed hold of the starched front of Sister V's habit and pulled it off. Sister V recoiled with a shocked look on her face. She certainly wasn't expecting that. She covered herself up and ran away in mortification. If she was clever she would have looked upon that incident as a valuable lesson. You can't abuse people and then hide behind your nun's habit, and use God's name to frighten children into behaving as you want them to. The girls locked themselves in the dormitory and refused to come out for Mass and lessons. After a couple of days they gave up because of hunger and they were punished and one of them was expelled and sent home. Shortly after this incident Sister V left St John's, none of the girls knew where she went.

One day recently, I was messing about in the shed at the bottom of our garden when my wife Diana entered with a piece of paper. She said that I had just received a fax from a lady who had read my book Deafness of the Mind and was at St John's at the same time as me. Her name was Maria. I cast my mind back to the 1940s at St John's trying to remember. Her name was familiar, but I couldn't remember what she looked like, which was not very surprising because in those far-off years at St John's the boys and girls were kept strictly segregated and not allowed to talk or even look at each other, and if caught doing so were punished for it. I think that they copied St John's when they built the Berlin Wall. Maria said in the fax that she hated every minute that she was there. She agreed with everything that I had said about the abuse and cruelty that was commonplace in those years, and it was about time that the truth was told. She would like to tell me the story about her time at St John's. I went to Leeds to see Maria so that she could tell me her story face to face. This is what she told me.

Maria was born in 1933 in Bradford, West Yorkshire. She was deaf at birth. At the tender age of 30 months she was sent to a school for deaf children in Bradford. It was common practice in those days to take deaf children away from their families, some children were taken from their families as young as two years of age and put into deaf and dumb Institutions. Maria has only vague memories of her stay at the deaf school in Bradford, after all she was only a little girl not yet three years of age. Her real memories began when she was aged five in 1938 and was sent to St John's. Her parents thought it would be better for her to be at St John's because she had an elder sister who was also deaf and in residence there, and so she would have someone to look after her.

I know from my own experience at St John's that the environment was cold and terrifying for little kids. Some of the Sisters were very cruel and sadistic. Not all of them were, some were nice, but as far as I knew these nice ones never said a word against the cruelty, or tried to put a stop to all the bullying and abuse that was going on there. Maybe they were too scared to say anything, or maybe they thought it was the normal thing to do, after all it was happening in other deaf institutions in Britain, and from what I was to learn later, it was happening to blind children in blind Institutions too. It seemed to me that they were trying to make us reject God for some reason. I got the impression that some of the Sisters were very bitter, but I refused to allow these people to come between me and my faith. I suppose that it makes a sick kind of sense. If a person has these cruel, sadistic impulses, where are the best places for them to gratify their sick urges? In Institutions for the deaf or blind children, of course.

Little Maria was soon to discover that behind the closed doors of the institution it was a very different world from the one her parents thought she was entering. It was a world that was full of bullying, lies, abuse and victimisation. Once in the classroom Maria was shocked to see the teacher, Sister V, pick up a thick heavy book and in a fit of temper bang one of the little girls on the head with it. The poor girl was nearly knocked unconscious and later suffered from a very bad headache. Another time the same Sister V took another little girl into a room where no one could see and made her stand on some steps to raise her up high enough so that she could cane her on her legs. The poor girl's legs were covered in black and blue welts. She showed her legs to Maria and told her what had happened. This is the same Sister V who had problems with other girls a few years later. These are just two of the many awful incidents that Maria was to witness.

It was indeed a very scary place for little deaf children. How on earth these children could be expected to believe in a good and merciful God when there were such sly, cruel monsters in Sisters' habits pretending to be good and holy in charge of them. Luckily for little Maria, at the outbreak of war in 1939 her father was in the army was stationed at Boston Spa. Very few people knew during the war that there was an ordnance factory making bombs and ammunition at nearby Thorpe Arch. Her Father was manning an anti-aircraft gun in one of the fields in the surrounding locality, and so he was able to visit his little daughter every day. That surely made Sister V think twice before she laid a heavy hand on little Maria.

When Maria was thirteen she and five other girls decided to run away. Where would they run away to? They had no idea, but they were so sick of all the relentless mental, emotional and physical torture and the endless praying they were forced to go. In their desperation, they just had to get away from that unnatural environment, if only for a short time. I can imagine just how they felt because I and two other lads had tried to run away too, but we didn't get very far. So one day they set off through the field at the back of the Institution and made their way to the river. Why did they decide to go there? Maria has no idea, they just did it. The river Wharfe could be very dangerous, it was very deep in places and with the eddies and whirlpools it was not the sort of place where children could play safely, but they didn't know that. Just to have that feeling of freedom away from the everlasting watchful gaze of the Sisters was wonderful. They ran and fooled about and had a great time, but in her mind Maria knew that eventually they had to go back to St John's and face the music, there was no other place they could go to.

While they were playing about, one of the girls slipped and fell into the river. This shocked them and made them realise that they had better go back and face the Sisters' wrath. So after pulling the unfortunate girl out of the river, which was not deep at that spot, they made their reluctant and fearful way back to St John's. As they entered through the front door, they were met with pandemonium. The Sisters were dashing about in a panic, searching everywhere for them. They were given a very severe talking to by Sister Magdalene and sent to bed with no supper, but luckily they were not caned, maybe because the summer holidays were only a couple of weeks away and they didn't want them to have any bruises or other evidence of ill-treatment when they went home.

During the school holidays Maria found a letter in the drawer at home. It was from Sister Magdalene and addressed to her mother. She asked her mother if she could read it. Her Mother said OK, go ahead. Sister Magdalene wrote that Maria had been a very bad girl, she had run away from school and had fallen in the river and was very lucky not to have drowned. Maria told her Mother that it wasn't true, she didn't fall in the river, it was another girl who fell in and the river was only about two foot deep at the place she fell in. Sister Magdalene was telling lies. Maria's Mother believed her, not Sister Magdalene.

Leaving St John's at the age of 16 with just one qualification for religious knowledge, Maria found employment as a clothing machinist in Leeds. At first, like most deaf school leavers, Maria was very shy and lacked self-confidence. She couldn't have any conversations with hearing people, or interact with them in any way because she had been shut away from the hearing world for so long, from 1938 to 1949, eleven long years incarcerated at St John's. It was almost like being in prison and her only crime was being deaf. On leaving St John's her head was filled with religious dogma and not one lesson on how to cope in the hearing world. It was many years before she had gained enough confidence to come out of her shell and interact with hearing people, Maria now has many hearing friends and lives quietly by herself after her beloved husband had passed away. Also on leaving St John's, Maria found that she was not so close to her family as she had been as a little girl. She had been away from them for far too long, like many other deaf children. Because of the long separation from their families they had the feeling that they had been abandoned. They were alienated from them; they had become strangers to their own families.

It was indeed a very lonely and isolated world for deaf people in those days. Most of them were taken away from their families at a very tender age, many never knowing a mother's love, never having a mother to cuddle them or tuck them in bed and kiss them goodnight. Instead they had the Sisters. It is possible that it made some deaf people harder, but many were badly affected by living in such an environment. Thankfully, those cruel days are long over, it is all in the past now, or is it really? There are far too many deaf people who were tortured for years with nightmares, which was the aftermath of their upbringing in those institutions. I think that this is something that the church and educational authorities should be ashamed of. They should apologise and beg forgiveness from the deaf community for the callous way in which they were treated. And I hope that we will never see such days again.

Many of the Sisters had been at St John's for many years. They had grown old there and during my time there about four of them had died in the Institute. Whenever that happened it was a macabre custom that the children had to go to the Sister's room where she was laid out in full habit and we had to look at the body and say a prayer and pay our last respects to the dead Sister. It was a scary experience and many of the boys had nightmares about it for weeks after. Some of the bigger boys would take the opportunity to scare the life out of the little ones by telling them stories of how the dead Sisters turned into bats and came at night when they were asleep to suck their blood, so the little ones would try to keep awake for as long as possible. The whole school had to attend the requiem Mass and after that we had to follow the procession to the cemetery and watch the coffin being lowered into the ground. Even the infants had to attend.

In 1951, when I had left St John's, my sister Patricia worked wonders on me. With the help of an old hearing aid she taught me how to pronounce words correctly, and to read and write better. She used her own homework from the convent where she was being educated by the Sisters. They must have been a lot different from the Sisters at St John's. Surely this underlines the difference in treatment between the hearing and deaf children. It clearly shows that we deaf children of the 1940s were the lost generation. Patricia's lessons must have sunk into my thick head, or maybe it was because I was learning in a better environment, because I seemed to be improving week by week, which made me think that with the right dedicated teachers any deaf child could receive a good education, even the children who were born deaf.

If only they had been allowed to use their own sign language, instead of this ridiculous oral system, which seemed to me to be not unlike teaching parrots to speak, but not with the same results. Parrots could speak better than many deaf kids. I have been told by some deaf friends that I was wrong to compare their reading and writing abilities at the age of sixteen to a hearing eight year old. They said that a hearing eight year old child was too far advanced on them, even when they were older than sixteen years, so they had a lot of catching up to do after their so-called education. Like most deaf people their education began after they had left school, but many never really caught up with their education after leaving school, I have labelled them 'The Lost Generations'.

I missed my wonderful sister Patricia when she emigrated to Canada at the age of 18 to be with her boyfriend. For a long time afterwards my eyes would well up whenever I thought of her and I hated that bloody Arthur Travis (her boyfriend) for taking her away. She had a good life when she moved to America; she married and had three lovely children. Tragically, she died of cervical cancer when she was in her early fifties. Rest in Peace Patricia, my lovely little blue-eyed blonde sister, you will always be a part of me, I will always be grateful to Patricia for her patience and understanding when teaching me to read and instilling in me a love of reading and books.

Reaching for the Stars

*A morsel of genuine history is a thing so rare
as to be always valuable*
Thomas Jefferson - third President of the United States

KEV! SURELY YOU can remember the good fun times you had with your old friends and move on now. Alright, I'll try to put those bad thoughts out of my mind. Let's forget St John's for the present. Let's go back to when I was 21 years old in 1956. I had just left my job working as a cutter for a Ladies' tailors and started working for the Ruberoid Roofing Company, who had their office and depot on Warwick Road, a few yards away from Manchester United's football ground. I had been given the address of this company by a deaf friend, Peter Kilgour, who used to work for them. Certainly from what Peter told me I could earn much more money in the roofing trade than I could as a cutter in a clothing factory, £15 as compared to £5. In the 1950s £15 a week was a good wage, and by the time I had left the roofing trade in 1990 the average wage for a roofer on some of the large sites was over £500 a week - roofing was far more interesting too.

In the summer of 1956, when applying for a job in the roofing trade, Mr. Birtles, the manager of the Ruberoid Roofing Company, had told me to report on Monday morning to Bob Doyle, the gaffer (foreman) at the building site in Trafford Park where a massive new warehouse was being built for the Senior Service tobacco company. The hourly rate would be 3s 9d an hour for a 60 hour week and all the overtime that we could handle, time and half for working on Saturday and double time for Sunday, which would boost our pay packets, riches indeed. There was no filling out of application forms, no CVs or anything like that, no questions about past experience, just, "Are you fit?" "Yes! Ok then, bring your P45, that's all." I must have been very lucky and fell in with a great gang of lads.

I will explain here before I get too deep into the story. In my opinion lip reading is not as great as some people would have you believe. It has its drawbacks: people are not always facing you when talking, they move their heads about and sometimes cover their mouths, chew gum or smoke cigarettes. When several people are talking it's very hard for a deaf person to follow the conversation, at least it is for me. Unless they are face to face lip readers can only pick up random words here and there. Also many words have the same mouth shape and usually the deaf person has to fill in the gaps by using his imagination, following the context of the conversation as seen by him/her and reading body language and facial expressions, which many deaf people are expert at and more often than not they are correct in their interpretation of the topic being discussed. Often the facial expression and body language will tell a truer story than the spoken word.

A very simple example of facial and body language telling the truer story is when someone has an accident, which happened a lot in the roofing trade. People will gather around gawping and someone will ask the inane question, "Are you alright?" The poor bloke's face will be contorted in agony, one leg may be sticking out at an unnatural angle, maybe his head split open and blood everywhere, but to the question "Does it hurt?" he will mutter through gritted teeth, "Nah! I'm ok, ahhh! Oh the pain! Yeah! I'm alright, Ahhh, be careful don't touch it" It's obvious to all and sundry that he is not alright, of course. Many times reading facial expressions and body language is much more subtle that this example, but I'm sure that you get the idea. The problem is lip reading is so tiring on your eyes, and the deaf person can't expect all hearing people to be facing him all the time, can he? That is why I much prefer to watch their mannerisms and the look on their faces as there are many clues as to what they are saying there. Anyway, words tend to have a hypnotic effect after trying to lip read for any length of time. And so by using these methods, lip reading and lots of guesswork following the context of conversations, combined with the help of a young lad called Wilf, who elected himself my "Official" interpreter, I am able to tell my story.

When I reported to Bob Doyle that warm summer morning, he muttered something I couldn't understand, I said, "Excuse me Mr. Doyle, I am deaf and I would like you to face me so that I can lip read you." I certainly caught the meaning of his next words. He exploded, "Aaahh! Fu^%#@$G, Bloody, bas*&^D sodding hell! Now they're scraping the bottom of the barrel, sending me this f**&%^g rubbin' rag." Then he stormed off muttering and cursing and waving his arms about and kicking things out of his way. I was taken aback by this outburst as there was no need for it. Bob Doyle was a big man of generous proportions, but I was as strong as a horse and could hold my own against anyone; I am an easy going, relaxed sort of bloke, but I could feel the anger starting to build up inside me. I went off after him shouting, "Hey you, come here fatty! Let's sort this out now, who the f+&*k do you think you are, talking to me like that, come back here you fat sod!" He just carried on storming off.

Before I could catch up with him one of the men grabbed hold of my arm and pulled me to one side. He said, "'Ere mate, Tak nae mind o' im, 'is bark is worse than 'is bite, 'e's like that wi' everyone the noo, e's under a lot 'o stress, 'e doan' mean it, ye come wi' me and I'll show ye what to do." At least that's what I thought he said! It was hard for me to understand his soft Scottish burr, but his body language and facial expression told me a lot of what he meant and I've made many of those words up myself.

At this time there were no steel scaffolding poles, wooden poles and ladders were used on building sites in Britain, and wire was used to lash everything together. Former seamen were favoured by the employers for scaffolding work because of their knowledge of knots. It may seem primitive to modern-day builders, but that method had been successfully used for hundreds, maybe thousands of years. Besides, we had not long come out of a war and steel was still rather scarce. Steel scaffold tubes gradually came into use in the late 1950s, early 1960s, when the SGB (Scaffolding Great Britain) company set up their business in the Manchester area and soon the use of steel scaffolding spread all over Britain. Sometime in the 70s aluminium scaffold tubes were tried because they were much lighter than the steel tubes and just as strong, but they all soon disappeared and ended up in scrapyards and that idea was discontinued.

The man who had pulled me away from Bob Doyle was of medium size, with blonde hair and a wispy blonde beard and moustache. He wore his beret on his head at a jaunty angle, and it only needed a feather on it and he would have been quite a dashing bloke, not unlike Errol Flynn in 'The Master of Ballantrae'. He introduced himself: "Ok mate, dinna fash thysel baht Bob, he'll be ok later, by t'way I'm Jock Locke, what's your name?" "I'm Kevin Fitzgerald," I said and we shook hands. Jock said, "I'll introduce ye to t'lads later on, just follow me for now." We approached the scaffolding and wooden ladder. I looked up and saw that there were three of these pole ladders lashed together to enable it to reach the top of the scaffolding. It all looked decidedly unsafe to me, Jock saw the dubious look on my face and said, "It's alright Kev, it's quite safe, just follow me and do what I do, if you hear a creaking noise like this, 'ccrreeeeaaak!' that's a warning that it is going to snap, so get off quick." Then he went scrambling up it like a monkey before I could explain to him that I was deaf and couldn't hear if it creaked like that. He practically ran up it, and when he reached the middle of the ladder it was bending alarmingly. It was swaying in and out with the motion of Jock as he ran up it and looked very unsafe. Jock reached the top and stepped onto the scaffold platform, looked down and saw me hesitating and shouted and gestured down, "Come on Kev, it's alright, it's safe, just do what I do." He beckoned me to come up, but the last time I had climbed up a ladder was in 1945 at St John's Boston Spa, when I had helped Mr. Harker the carpenter to fix the broken window in the girls' bathroom, and what a caning I had for it! That was only a few feet high, but this was a different matter; this was about one hundred feet high. It was frightening, and so with some trepidation I put my foot on the first rung and thus began my 34-year career as a roofer.

At first going up that ladder was alright, but when I got halfway up the swaying motion became worse and though I wasn't able to hear any creaking, I was confident that I would certainly feel if it was going to snap. When I reached the middle the swaying was worse; I was holding on for dear life. I couldn't move, it was terrifying. A grizzled old man with a leathery weather-beaten face who was coming up below me touched me on the leg. I looked down at him and he was making a shooing gesture and saying, "It's ok kid, just take it one rung at a time, it's quite safe." It seemed to me that they were rather fond of saying "It's quite safe" when to my eyes it looked anything but "safe".

So with my heart in my mouth, I had a last look around at the world that I had suddenly decided I loved very much and didn't want to leave just yet. I put one foot after the other in time to the swaying of the ladder and made ready to leap off on to the scaffolding at the slightest suspicion of the ladder snapping in half. Finally I reached the top and stepped off onto the scaffolding platform with a sigh of relief and a silent prayer of thanks to my Guardian Angel. However, my relief was short-lived because Jock then picked up a metal 8ft x 4ft roofing sheet from a pile that was on the scaffold. "Git one o' them Kev an' foller me," he said. Then he nonchalantly stepped onto the steel girder and carried it across to the other side about 40 feet away. The steel H girder was about 12 inches wide and 24 inches deep. I bent forward and looked down. I could see there was a drop of about 90 feet or so to the ground, which was a mass of rubble, bricks, lumps of broken concrete, planks etc. There was no chance of surviving a fall from that height on to that. I was trying to swallow but my throat had suddenly gone dry. The leathery-faced old man, who I later learned was Albert Mason, said, "It's ok kid, it's quite safe, take it steady and watch where you put your feet." No way was I going to carry a steel roofing sheet across that chasm on a 12 inch-wide girder. I could see that the other men who had come up the ladder behind us were having a chuckle about my predicament. Now I can't allow that, can I eh? So I sat down astride the girder with the sheet across it in front of me. I told myself, "Don't look down Kev", then I pushed the sheet forward, then slid forward on my bum, and so push, slide, push, slide I made my way across. When I reached the other side all the lads gave me a cheer. It was like I had passed some kind of test.

Later on, when thinking back to that scenario on that first day and wondering why they had dropped me in at the deep end like that, something clicked in my mind and I understood that is how they got rid of people who had no head for heights. They must have been expecting me to give up and go home. Did they think that because I was deaf and new to roofing I couldn't do the job? Was Bob Doyle's attitude to me on that first meeting a kind of test too? They didn't know about the great incentive I had to stick with this job. I wanted to earn enough money to marry Diana and make a home and family with her, and for that reason they wouldn't get rid of me so easily. I didn't know at the time that my deafness was affecting my balance; I just thought that I had to focus hard, just like everybody else had to do. I think that in those days even doctors didn't know that deafness can affect your balance, or if they did then nobody told me about it. I know that many of my deaf friends who had been stopped by the police because they were not walking straight, and when made to walk a straight line to prove that they were not drunk were unable to do so, had to spend some time in the police station until the Deaf Missioner could come and explain to the police. Such was the ignorance in the larger hearing population about matters concerning the deaf. The phrase 'Deaf Awareness' had not been coined in those days.

In the 1950/60's most jobs that paid a decent wage were closed to deaf people, bench joinery, shoe repairing and the clothing trade seemed to be the only jobs that would accept deaf people. I remember a story going around at the time about two deaf men who found jobs working for a road resurfacing company. Their job was to control the flow of traffic. They would stand on each end of the road where the work was going on with these signs on a pole, rather like the ones lollipop ladies have, one side was red with the word 'STOP' the other side was green with the word 'GO'. All went well as long as they could see each other, but when they were working on a bend in the road and couldn't see each other then they had problems. It sometimes descended into a Laurel and Hardy farce, with both the deaf men showing 'GO' or 'STOP' at the same time as they were unable to see each other. Traffic was meeting in the middle, and sometimes some awkward drivers refused to back up and screaming and yelling at each other ensued. As you can imagine, they didn't last long in that job. I think that after one colossal mix up where drivers were exchanging blows our heros thought it better to disappear and so went home.

We were constantly coming up against barriers and brick walls in our quest to find a good job. Many deaf people were only allowed to do the most menial jobs, even criminals just out of prison and drug addicts were treated better than the average deaf person. As the average hearing man wouldn't take on a job such as roofing, with all its inherent risks, I suppose the Ruberoid Roofing Company was happy to have a strong lad like me working for them.

When I explained to the lads that I was deaf they just made light of it. Jock said, "Aw mon, that's nowt, lookit auld Albert there, 'e's got a gammy right arm. I looked and sure enough his arm was held against his side and his fingers were drawn into his hand like hooks, unable to be opened or closed into a fist. He looked as if he had something wrong with one of his eyes too. His left eye had a heavy eyelid, it was half way down and it covered half of his eye pupil. I couldn't believe it, how on earth does he get up a ladder that swayed as much as that one with only one arm? Jock said, "Lookit auld Stan there, 'e's allbut blind, he can only see about three feet in front o' hissel". "Good Heavens!" I replied, "Are they safe to work at heights like this?" "Yeah! Course they are," Jock answered casually, "They're in their 60s the noo and they've been in this trade a' their lives, they may as well stay 'til they retire noo, nowt else they can do. There was also a man called Peter who had only a forefinger and thumb on his right hand and he could pinch as hard as a pair of pliers. You gotta be a wee bit crazy to be a roofer, but the money is good, more than the brickies and joiners and other 'safe' trades can earn." Blimey! I wondered what on earth I had let myself in for. With men like these it's no wonder we won the war. The Nazis and Japanese didn't stand a chance against men like these. They all had hard as iron bodies and thick hands and fingers, so better to be friends with them I told myself.

We spent the rest of the day fixing the roofing sheets to the steel purlins nearly 100 feet up above Trafford Park, which at that time was the largest industrial estate in Europe, maybe in the world. During the war Trafford Park was one of the main targets for the German Luftwaffe bombers, so there was a lot of re-building work to be done there. Maybe that is one of the reasons why they were willing to overlook the fact that I was deaf and gave me a job. Except for the part where I had to ascend and descend that rickety ladder and walk across that steel, I quite enjoyed working up there above all the noise and bustle. Sometimes, when the wind was from the right direction, I could see for miles. On a clear day I could even see the Welsh mountains in the distance, other times the view was obscured by the smoke from the factory chimneys. It was hard in winter, and sometimes in freezing weather I wished that I was anywhere else but on a roof with my icy hands trying to fasten the nuts and bolts. In those situations a hot sweet mug of tea was always welcome. I wondered if this is why people climbed mountains. It was very different from working in a clothing factory; I thought, "Yeah! I'm going to like this. I'll have to take the bad with the good," and on the whole there were more good days than bad days.

Did I tell you there was no Health and Safety Commission in those days; people were responsible for their own safety. Today it would be impossible for a deaf man to get a job as a roofer, which I think is very unfair. In all my years working on big and small roofing jobs I never had a serious accident, though I saw many bad accidents, even deaths, involving hearing people. Nowadays, with the Health and Safety Commission inspecting every site and laying down rules, there are just as many accidents and deaths as there were in the old days. According to them deaf people can't even have jobs sweeping the streets because they can't hear traffic behind them, so with today's young deaf people there is a culture of living on benefits, which is a shame. The health and safety people have taken away their pride. I had to be much more careful and concentrate far more than the other lads, who seemed, in my opinion, to treat the job far too casually. They were too ready to say "It's quite safe" when one wrong step could send them plummeting to the ground. Maybe they were just showing off and it was all bravado, but that is how accidents happen.

Somehow I got through that first day as a roofer. When I got home that evening mam was waiting for me with a worried expression on her face, and a big plate of tater hash. She said, "I put two cow heels in that Kevin, you're going to need a lot of food now that you're working outside on building sites." I was starving so I tucked into my dinner with gusto, I felt like Desperate Dan of comic fame and his cow pie, so I had a second helping too. Mam looked at my dirty weather-beaten face and said, "Oh, Kevin, why don't you go back to the clothing factory? You were clean and safe there." "Don't worry Mam," I told her, "I'll be ok, they are a great bunch of lads and they will look out for me."

Next morning, on waking up I thought I would jump out of bed in my usual way, but I was as stiff as a board. I had aches and pains all over from the unaccustomed hard work, and the fact that I had to keep focused when I was up on top was very tiring too. I hobbled painfully downstairs to where mam had our breakfast ready. As I was eating my porridge, mam put an old army bag down beside my chair and said, "I've put you some ham butties in there Kevin, and an old brew can of your Dad's with some tea and sugar." "Thanks Mam," I shouted as I dashed out to catch the early morning bus to Trafford Park. As I walked onto the site I was greeted by a different Bob Doyle. There was a beaming smile spread across his round weather-beaten face. He walked over to me and put his mouth right up against my ear and bellowed at the top of his voice, which reverberated all round the building site, "Top o' t'morn t' ye me lad, how are ye feelin' this fine summer's morning?" I flinched away from him. "I'm alright, bit stiff but ok. Please, there's no need to shout like that, just face me when talking and I will lip read you," I replied. "Oh Good!" He bellowed. "I want you down here on the ground today." Phew! I breathed a sigh of relief. I'll be working on terra firma today. "We are going to insulate and cover those steel sheets we put on yesterday, make it all water tight, and I want you to give Old Len the pot man a lift with the bitumen, Ok?" "Ok! Got it Mr. Doyle." "Ah, lad! Just call me Bob. There's the pots and Len is over there, now off you go me lad." He was still bellowing at the top of his voice, he must have had a naturally loud voice, and it must have been the reason why he was the foreman, as he sure was a forceful character.

What Bob had called pots turned out to be three rather massive big coal-fired boilers on wheels in which the melted bitumen was bubbling away like a witch's evil brew. It was a really scary sight, black bubbles were working their way up from the dark depths of the boilers and spewing out a yellow sulphorous stinking gas as they burst on the surface. Len was in charge of them and he had to be there at the crack of dawn to light the boilers and get everything ready for the roofers. This was before the days of propane gas canisters and coal was used and so it took some time to heat up the bitumen to a working temperature. Len was about 50 years old, not a tooth left in his head, which had a wild uncombed tangle of wiry grey hair. Also, he had a slim and wiry build and was of average height with weather-beaten features and a large squashed pockmarked nose, and, as I found out later, he was deceptively strong. His job had given him scrawny whipcord muscles and the sinews and tendons stuck out on his arms, which seemed to me to be more sinew than muscle.

As I approached him he stopped me by holding his hand out like a policeman stopping traffic, then he shouted across the building site to someone and beckoned him over. I saw Wilf coming towards us, and when Wilf arrived he and Len talked together for a few minutes. Then Wilf said to me that Len wanted him to interpret what he was saying because his Lancashire dialect was very broad, and he wanted to make sure that I understood him. I wanted to add that it would be very hard to lip read him as he had no teeth, but I kept quiet. And so through Wilf, Len greeted me with "'Ello lad," and then he said, "'Av ye got a ciggy fer me?" I spoke direct to Len: "Sorry Len, I don't smoke." Then through Wilf Len said, "AArr! Bloody 'ell, ne'er ye mind now lad! I want ye to respect this hot stuff, ye maunt mess wi' it, careful pourin' it in t' deggers, it can cause ter-r-r-rible burns. Do what I tell ye an' ye'll be alright lad. If ye do spill some on yersel' run to t' yon tap, see it there up t' broo an' stick it under." He pointed to a standpipe some yards away. "OK lad?" Wilf made an excellent job of copying Len's dialect and idioms; he was mimicking Len, even the way he spoke. Daft innit! Wilf and I had a good laugh about it afterwards. "Ok Len! Under the tap quickish," I said. Len said (through Wilf), "Right! Now see yon lads pullin' those boxes of insultin' (Insulation) boards up?" I looked over to where Len was pointing and two lads were pulling up a cardboard box by means of a rope and gin wheel, and there was a pile of boxes nearby waiting to be pulled up. "When I fill a degger with this hot bitumen I want ye to take it over to 'em, they will pull it up, but first ye mun clear a path through a' this rubble, ye caunt be carrying hot bitumen o'er it, it's too dodgy see, an' while yer at it me lad, keep yer eyes open fer me fawse teef, I cannae remember where I pu' 'em." I found out that a degger was also a metal three gallon can with a pouring spout which was placed on some bricks with a coal fire under it and filled with water for brewing tea, all very Spartan, but we were not fussy. (I hope you can understand this Lanky dialect of Len's, I've done my best to get it right.)

When I took the first degger of hot bitumen over to the lads pulling up the boxes, I looked up and saw that old Albert was taking them off. He was holding on to the scaffold pole with his good arm and leaning out so that he could reach the rope with his bad arm, which he couldn't fully straighten out. He would hook his bad hand round the rope and pull it and the box onto the scaffold. I thought, "This is crazy, I don't want to be anywhere near here when they pull the deggers of boiling hot bitumen up," but I found out later that Albert never spilled a drop and everyone trusted him. I was told by one of the lads that years before Albert was on a roof that collapsed under him and sent him plummeting to the ground. That's how he lost the use of his right arm. After a few days Len and I were able to dispense with Wilf's services as by that time I had got used to Len's way of speaking, and I had taught him a few simple signs and gestures, so we got along very well. The word must have spread through the Manchester Mafia (See below) about Len and me and how we could understand each other, while others who could hear perfectly couldn't understand him, because a few years in the future when I was working for a different company, there was a lad who had a very bad stutter and people found it hard to understand him, so the bosses in their wisdom thought, "Well, here is a lad who can't hear, and here is a lad who can't speak, let's put them working together and see what happens. If Kev could understand old Len then he should have no problem with this one." What happened was that Ted (the lad's name) and I got on very well after I taught him a few signs and gestures and we worked together for a while.

The first few weeks in the roofing trade were so different from anything I had ever experienced before that they have stuck in my mind. I can remember those first weeks so vividly. Later on, as I became used to working on roofs, I developed a laser-like concentration to make up for my poor sense of balance. I found that if I was holding something, a hammer, drill etc., it helped me to focus better. I think that when I lost my hearing, another sense compensated and would be fine-tuned to make up for the loss of my hearing, but I still had to focus fiercely. It's all about Mind over Matter.

The Manchester Mafia

The great end of life is not knowledge but action
Thomas Henry Huxley

NOTHING WOULD SHOCK me like those first few weeks as a roofer. I found it different from anything I had ever experienced before. I found that the roofers had what I can only describe as a "Roofers' code". It was not the done thing to talk about any accidents you may have had, especially about burns from hot bitumen. Many of the men had bad scars from burns, so they didn't need to talk about it, the evidence was there for all to see. In those days only the Jessie boys wore protective gloves, which they had to provide themselves. I was one of the 'Jessie boys' and I didn't care who knew it. Another thing I found out was what they called the 'Manchester Mafia'. Every roofer in Manchester and the surrounding area knew each other and it wasn't long before they all knew about 'Deaf Kev'.

I had to join the union, the EEPTU, the Electrical, Engineering & Plumbing Trades Union. The monthly union meetings in the Wheatsheaf pub in Manchester often developed into mammoth drinking sessions with roofers from other firms and I was introduced all round. I didn't have a clue what they talked about at these meetings. I would catch a snippet of information here and there and nodded my head wisely in agreement when I saw the others nodding their heads, and shook my head vehemently in disagreement when they did, but I enjoyed having a drink with the lads. Despite sinking many pints of bitter we all turned out for work bright and early and raring to go the next morning.

Being naturally inquisitive, one day while we were sat around the pot having a tea and cig break, I asked Bob about the origin of Built-Up Felt Roofing, or BUR roofing as it was known in the trade. I was told that it began in Belfast in the 19th century by a man named Anderson, who established the Anderson Red Hand Roofing Company. It was the first to marry felt and bitumen as roofing materials and use it especially for flat roofs. The Ruberoid Roofing Company started in Newcastle at about the same time or not long after Andersons. Sometime in the 1920s Ruberoid opened an office and depot on the corner of Warwick Road in Trafford Park near Manchester United's football ground and sent some men to get it started up, so that is why there were such a lot of Geordies working there, such as Jimmy Birtles, Tommy Bell, Billy Dryden, Bob Coulson, Jimmy Collins and Jock Farmer. I have to mention Jock even though he was a true Scot, not a Geordie, because he was one of the most colourful characters in the roofing trade, but one of the most difficult men for me to understand his speech. He often said that Englishmen were a mongrel race, and the only true British were the Scots, Welsh and Irish, but I was alright because my mam was Welsh and Dad was Irish so that made me Celtic. I thought that he should have brushed up on his history, but I said nothing, I wanted a peaceful life.

These Geordies were a dour lot who loved their pints followed by a malt whiskey, especially Tommy Bell. Old Bob Coulson was an ardent Manchester City fan, and every Saturday when 12 o'clock was near he would pack up his tools and tell us that he had to go to the office to sort out some problem. He would tell us that we had to stay on the job until four o'clock, then we could pack up and go home. He was fooling nobody as we all knew that he was off to the football match. As soon as he was safely round the corner and away we all packed up and went home. There were many other

great characters in the roofing trade whose names have long
disappeared into the mists of time. There was fierce rivalry
between Ruberoid Roofing and Andersons Roofing, both
firms claiming that they were the best roofing firms in Great
Britain.

At the annual Xmas 'Do' for Ruberoid roofers, after a
few pints and rousing renditions of 'The Blaydon Races',
many old scores were settled with roofers from other sites.
Sometimes it was like a scene from the films of the Wild
West where a brawl kicks off in the saloon. One of the lads
was called Eric Brown and he was only a little man, but he
used to be a lightweight boxing champion in the army and
he had the squashed nose to prove it. He told me that it was
best not to use your fists because the bones in your hand are
easily broken. That's why boxers always bandage their hands,
it's to protect their hands, not their opponents face. Eric
said, "Always use your head Kev." I thought, "Now, there's
a gentleman!" I assumed that he meant it is always best to
use your wits and talk your way out of trouble, until one day
when trouble flared up and I saw him put down two men
twice his size by jumping up and quick as a flash knee-jerked
into their groin and butted them in the face with his head.
That method of fighting was called 'The Liverpool Kiss', but
I suppose that in Liverpool they called it 'The Manchester
Kiss'. That's what Eric had meant by "Best to use your head
Kev". I was learning a lot here. The first lesson that Eric gave
me was that if ever I go to Liverpool I must keep my hands
down low protecting my 'vitals'. I thought that I would have
to walk about in Liverpool holding my wotsits, I was very
naïve then and I realised later that Eric was having a laugh at
my expense. These lads make wonderful friends, but terrible
enemies.

Another thing that I learned was they don't like people
who are too cocky and try to throw their weight around. These

men would not stand for it. So it was a very dangerous thing to be a bully on a building site as these lads wouldn't put up with it for long, especially on the roofs where a little nudge when on the edge, or some spilt boiling hot bitumen could so easily cause an 'accident'. I remember on one site where the gaffer was a big loud-mouthed bully, always shouting at and pushing the young lads, who were quite cowed by him. He was the opposite of Bob Doyle, who was a big man and had a very loud voice, but was no bully. You could always have a laugh with him, and he became a good friend of mine. This man, who shall remain nameless, was different. Anyway, on this particular day something happened that showed him the error of his ways. There was a young lad who took orders for fish and chips or whatever it was you fancied for your dinner. He also collected the tray of brew cans and mugs. He would brew up, leave the tray on the table, run to the chippy, get the orders, come back, put it all in the cabin then shout up, "Dinner's ready". All the lads came sliding down the ladders and sat down in their usual places, ate their dinners and drank their tea, and then they would light up their ciggies and have a game of cards or read the papers.

The nameless one would sit in the corner eating his dinner apart from the other men. He always had a scowl on his face, which tended to put people off trying to make conversation with him. These brew cans, which were common in those days, could hold three cups of tea. The cup was the metal lid of the brew can doing duty as a cup. We would hold the brew can by the handle and swing it round in a circle, and this would mix the tea, sugar and milk up nicely. He had already had two cups of tea and was pouring his third when he suddenly stopped. He must have made some strange gurgling noise, because everybody stopped what they were doing and turned to look at him. His face was ashen, his eyes were bulging, I thought he was having a heart attack or choking. Then one lad pointed to his cup. It seemed that when pouring the last cup of tea a dog turd had slipped out of the brew can onto the edge of the cup, half had gone into the cup and half had gone down the outside of it, leaving a brown smear down the side of the cup. Wow! That man had just drunk two cups of dog turd-flavoured tea and never noticed that it tasted funny. He jumped to his feet, with his face having taken on a greenish tinge, and pointed to his tea cup with a shaking finger. "What the bloody 'effin' 'ell is that?" he screamed. The young tea lad came over to him to see what the matter was and a mighty back-handed smack across his face sent him flying across the room. The nameless one then held his mouth and ran outside to spew it all up. We never found out who had put that dog turd into his brew can as nobody would admit to doing it, but that man had made a lot of enemies. He was moved to another building site after that and we were told that he had become very meek and mild. After witnessing that incident I was very, very careful to be nice to everybody, even the smallest ones - especially the smallest ones - on building sites. It is just as easy to be nice as to be nasty. Another lesson I had learned then: be warned, it certainly didn't pay to be nasty on building sites

It was a custom among roofers on some sites to sit around the bitumen pots when having a tea and cig break, or at dinner time if you were not inclined to go to the nearest pub. Even on the hottest Summer day you would find some of them sitting on bricks or upturned buckets around the pot, passing the time telling stories. Some men would bring potatoes and drop them in the pot of bubbling hot bitumen. The potatoes would sink to the bottom and after a few minutes rise to the top where they would be scooped out and left for a few minutes to cool sufficiently to have the bitumen peeled off and the lovely aroma of baked potatoes would fill the air. Many of these men were in the forces during the war and they had many interesting stories to regale us with. Bob Doyle with his parade ground voice was a sergeant in the Royal Marines, Jock Locke was in the Royal Navy and Hughie was in the Merchant Navy taking supplies to the Russians at Murmansk.

Charlie Hornsby told us that he was among the soldiers who liberated one of the concentration camps. He told us how sickened he was to see how badly the Nazis could treat fellow human beings. He said that he got hold of one of the camp guards, took him out of sight of anybody and beat him to within an inch of his life. He couldn't help himself, he was so angry. He took his watch, money and anything of value that he had on him and dragged him, slapping and kicking him all the way to the prison compound. In the end he had to be pulled off this guard. He said that the guard was smirking as if he was proud of what he had done, as if it was a good thing, and he seemed to think that I would agree with him and approve what had happened in those camps, so he just lost his temper and beat the stuffing out of him. Charlie said that those people don't deserve to be treated like fellow humans.

Another man I met was named Yan. I don't know if it was his real name but it was what they were calling him. Young Wilf explained to me that Yan was Polish and was a fighter pilot in the Battle of Britain. He always had a half pint bottle of vodka in his pocket and would take sips from it throughout the day, even when he was up on the steel, it seemed to steady his nerves. Many of these ex-forces men were finding it very difficult to settle down in peacetime, so roofing, with its element of danger, was an ideal job for them. Roofing was also the only job where I could earn decent wages and where I would be accepted and where my deafness didn't seem to matter to the lads. I met many interesting characters in the roofing trade, that's for sure.

When walking across Piccadilly one morning on my way to get the bus to work, there was a sudden very loud piercing noise that went right through my right ear and made the hair on my head stand up in spikes. A cat that was sleeping on a nearby wall suddenly jumped up screeching with its hair standing on end and a dog dashed off into the distance with its tail between its legs. I quickly covered my ear with my hand and looked round to see what it was. People were frozen into the positions they were in when the noise happened. In the distance I saw Bob Doyle, who was waving his arm at me and giving this piercing whistle. When I waived back he stopped whistling and yelled, "Ke e e vvviiin!" So I ran over to him as I thought the windows in the nearby buildings would shatter and he would be arrested if he didn't stop that noise. You must understand he is not like that normally. It was only because I am deaf and it was for my benefit. We caught the bus and travelled to work together.

These men were tough as old leather and as hard as iron, but many of them had a very childish sense of humour. One day a young lad came on the building site at Trafford Park. I happened to be down below at the time, so I had a grandstand view of what happened. This young lad must have been about 17 and he approached me and apprehensively asked for Mr. Doyle. Before I could answer him someone from on top bellowed down. Wilf told me later what had transpired and it went like this: "Oy you! Never mind 'im, he cannae hear ye, what do ye want?" The young lad replied timidly, "Please sir, the office sent me, I have to report to Mr. Doyle." "Mr. who?" "Please Sir, Mr. Doyle." "Nah! Don't know no Mr. Doyle on this site, wait a minnit I'll ask the lads. Hey fellers! anyone 'ere know Mr. Doyle?" "Doyle? Doyle? – oh! I think he means Fatty." "Oh yeah! That's right. Hey kid, nobody calls him Mr. Doyle, he's called Fatty, so just go over there. See that big man? That's him, just say, 'Hey fatty, the office has sent me'.

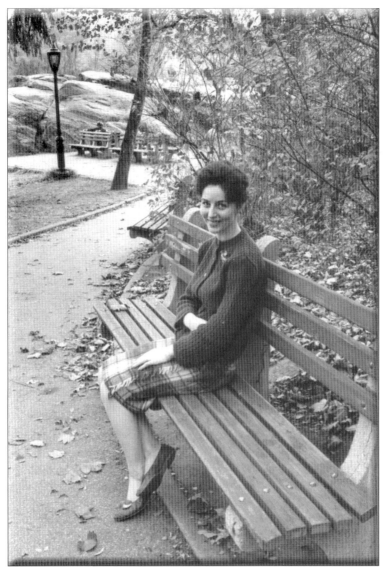

My sister Patricia pictured in Central Park, New York in 1961. She instilled in me a love of the English language. I was upset when she emigrated to Canada with her boyfriend when she was 18 in 1955.

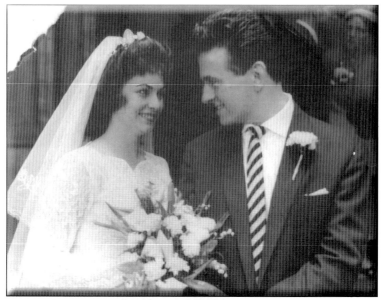

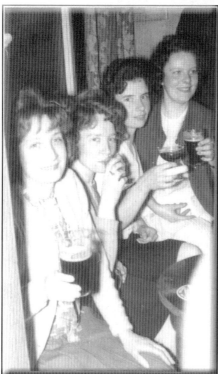

Diana and I married
in 1959 (above), which
left the girls from the
Liverpool Deaf Club
(left) broken-hearted.
This picture was taken
the night my friends
and myself had to walk
all the way back to
Manchester down the
East Lancs Road.

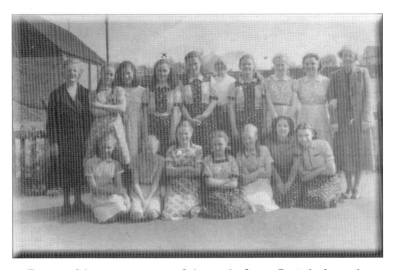

Pictured here are some of the girls from St. john's in the 1940s. Fourth from the left is Maria, who contacted me after the publication of Deafness of the Mind to tell me her harrowing experiences of St. John's.

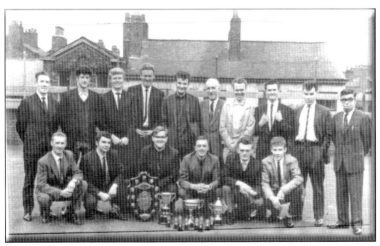

Pictured here are some of the members of Manchester Deaf Club in the 1960s with the trophies they had won for football and snooker. In the background in The Griffin pub, which still stands next to Manchester Royal Infirmary.

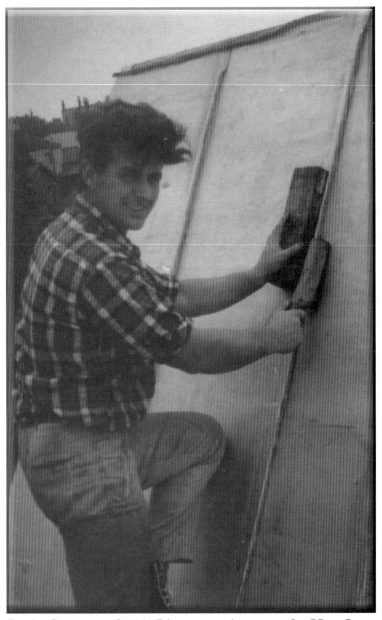

In the Summer of 1956 I began work as a roofer. Here I am pictured using my aerodynamic hairstyle to stay upright.

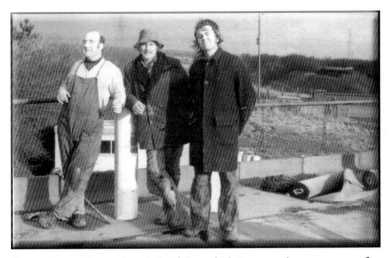

I am pictured on the right (above) doing my best to pose for the camera. On the left is Don Andrews, who ironically was scared of heights, and in the middle Hughie Chadwick.

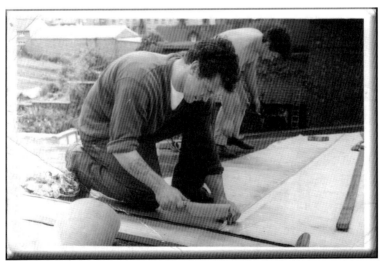

Bob O'Connor does his best to block me out of this photo. Roofing was a very dangerous occupation, particularly for someone who was deaf. I was lucky to never have a serious accident, although I witnessed many.

CHIEF EXECUTIVE
148 Old Street
LONDON
EC1V 9HQ

Telephone 0171 250 2888
Fax 0171 250 2960

18 June 1997

Mr Kevin Fitzgerald
543 Oldham Road
Middleton
MANCHESTER
M24 2DH

Dear Mr. Fitzgerald,

Thank you for your letter of 10th June 1997 and the copy of the letter you have sent to the Editor of Courier.

I was very sorry to hear that you felt there was bullying and discrimination. There is no place for either in The Post Office and I want to see everyone doing all they can to remove it.

You have had real success in achieving City and Guilds awards. I congratulate you on them and hope that they are proving to be of real practical value in the Manchester Mail Centre.

As I said in Bristol, to obtain such awards is a great achievement, made all the greater by the need to overcome a hearing disability. I hope that through the example of people like Sandra Small and yourself, we will be able to motivate other employees to take up this challenge.

Thank you for writing to me - I shall look forward to seeing your letter in Courier: and any replies.

Yours sincerely

John Roberts

JOHN ROBERTS CBE

The Post Office made a grudging acknowledgement
of my complaints about discrimination.

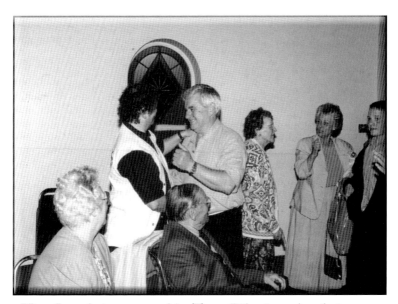

Here I am being greeted by Terry Riley jnr., the chairman
of the British Deaf Association (BDA) at my 60th birthday.
In the foreground seated are his mother and father whilst
Diana is deep in conversation in the middle of the three
ladies on the right.

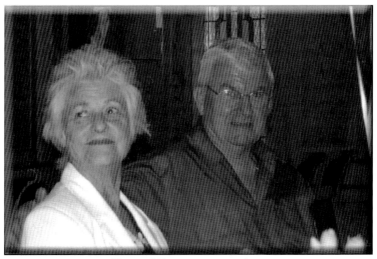

Di and I as we are today.

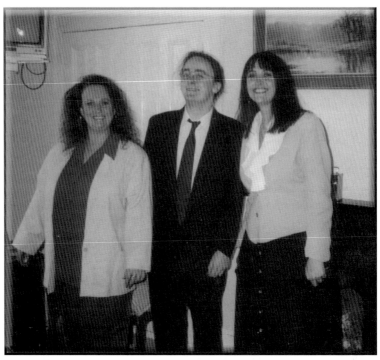

Above: Our children, Rosemary, John and Lynn.

Below: Di and I with our dogs, Fitzie and Sunny, and various grandchildren and great grandchildren. From the left: Scarlet, Megan, Georgia holding baby Talulah and Jack.

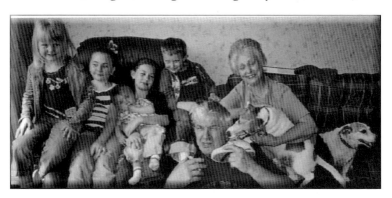

Go on, it's ok." The poor kid went over to Bob and said in all
innocence, "Hey fatty, the office has sent me." I could feel the
ground shaking when Bob roared, "Yer cheeky little monkey!,
Ahhh! just ye wait 'til I get me 'ands on yer." The kid ran for
his life. Luckily Bob looked up just then and saw the lads on
top of the scaffold rolling about in hysterics. He realised then
what had happened. Those lads were having a laugh, so he
shook his ham-like arm and massive fist at them, but it only
made them laugh all the more.

At this time, 1959, Diana and I were finally married in St
Cuthbert's Church in Withington. The reception was held in
the Midland Hotel, Withington and friends and family had a
great time. Then we caught the train to Fleetwood to get the
ferry to the Isle of Man for our two weeks honeymoon. Only
rich people could afford holidays abroad in the 1950s and
I was far from rich. When we came back to Manchester as
husband and wife, I was in a different world. I was a married
man now and I had responsibilities. I couldn't think just about
myself anymore. Here was a beautiful girl who depended on
me to look after her.

Diana's parents lived in a big five-bedroomed Victorian
house on Mauldeth Road West in Withington. Her mam
offered to let us stay and use the top floor as our flat to give us
the opportunity to save up for our own house. I thought that
was very good of them and accepted gladly. The house had
extensive cellars, so I asked Di's mam if I could use them as
a gym. She agreed, so I made some benches and power rack,
pulleys, got lots of weight plates and bars and started training
again. Very soon I had about six other lads training with me. I
soon became very strong and put more muscle on by following
Ken Latham's training methods. Every Wednesday after
work I would get the bus to Stockport where my pal Johnny
Glancy lived. He taught weight training and wrestling in the
evenings to young lads in one of the local schools and he had

asked me to help him. With all this activity, working on roofs, up and down ladders all day, coming home and training in the cellar, then helping Johnny Glancy in Stockport, I never became one of these very big body-builders, but I became very hard and strong and my appetite shot up sky high, I would think nothing about eating two roast chickens, lashings of vegetables, ice cream and my favourite custard cream biscuits. I was 5ft 7in and I weighed 13 and a half stone.

I worked hard and Diana saved up too and in 1963 we finally secured a mortgage on a three-bedroom semi-detached house in my old home town of Middleton. The vendor wanted £2,000 for the house, but I managed to get it reduced to £1,940 because the window frames were showing signs of rot and I would have to replace them. Just a few years later house prices shot up sky high and we were lucky to get our feet on the property ladder just in time. In those days there was no bonus system in the building trade. That came later, in the 1970s I think. In the 1950s and 60s we were paid for the hours we worked, plus time and half for working overtime and Saturdays and double time for working on Sundays, so as there was no bonus system it meant that we could take our time and do a good job. Thanks to Hitler's Luftwaffe there was lots of work to be done around Manchester.

One big job was at AV Roe's (later to become British Aerospace) factory in Chadderton near where I lived before I married. That factory was one of the main targets for German bombers because it was where the Lancaster bombers were made, and those British bombers were causing havoc to the German munitions factories. These Lancaster bombers, along with the American super fortresses, went a long way to winning the war for us.

Ruberoid roofs were guaranteed for 25 years, unlike today when they only guarantee the roofs for one year. They say that if there are any faults in the roof they will show up within a year, but really it's rubbish to say that. It was brought about by the new bonus system and using cheap shoddy materials. The lads were rushing the jobs to earn as much money as possible, so because of the rushing to complete the work, there was a lot of shoddy work that could no longer be guaranteed for 25 years. Back in the 1950s and 60s, if it was raining we stayed in the cabin, it was too dangerous to go up on top in bad weather, and the bitumen wouldn't stick to wet surfaces, so we played cards, etc. There was no rush at all, but all that changed when the new bonus system came in. Thursday was when Bob Doyle gave us our wages. He came from the office with a big wad of notes and a bag of change. We would go into the cabin one by one while he counted out our money, which we signed for against our names on a slip of paper.

One day one of the men called George came in to work with his head and back of his neck swathed in bandages. We asked him what had happened, and he explained to us that the previous day, a pay day, it had been raining all day and his wages were burning a hole in his pocket, so he joined the lads playing poker and had a streak of bad luck. He just kept losing his money but kept telling himself that his luck was bound to change soon. Besides, he had to win some money back as his wife would go mad when she found out how much he had lost, so he carried on playing, praying that his luck would change. He just had to recoup some money. One hour later he was down to his last pound note out of his £20 wages, for which he had worked hard for seven days to earn. He had to leave the game and get the bus home, all the way home to Middleton on the number 17 bus. He was thinking how to explain to his wife where all his wages had gone, and dreading that moment.

Alighting from the bus in Middleton, he put his hand into his pocket and pulled out 7/6d, which was all he had left to see his wife and two kids through the week. He was thinking of telling his wife that he had been mugged and his wages were stolen, but he doubted if she would believe him, George was a big, weather-beaten, formidable looking bloke, not the sort of man muggers would dare to risk picking on. He was trying to think of how to put off the dreaded moment when he would have to explain to his wife where all his wages had gone. Then, as he turned the corner into Wood Street, he saw the bookies. The sign over the door was beckoning to him very enticingly. He thought, "I might as well, I've got nothing to lose now, only my life if the favourite doesn't win." So giving way to temptation, he opened the door and went in.

Inside the bookies doorway there was a shallow well where a coconut-fibre mat usually lay, but it was not there on this particular day. On entering George tripped on the edge of the well, caught his shoe on it and ripped the sole of his shoe so that it flapped as he walked. "AARRH! That's all I f(*&^g well need." He growled like a bear with a sore head as he flapped his way to the counter and put his last money on the favourite, which true to form came fifth. George just wasn't having any luck at all; the fates were all conspiring against him that day. He turned away in despair, dreading to go home and face his wife. Now, it must be understood that George was a big man and not scared of any man, but his wife, well that was a different matter. She was formidable woman too, though she was a tiny woman. She had been known to put some men in hospital for getting too familiar and slighting her. She could turn into a screeching, scratching hellcat in the blink of an eye.

Just as our George was leaving the bookies a rolls royce pulled up and the bookie, Gus Greenstein, got out. He was dressed in a flash pin-striped suit, tan camel hair overcoat, gold and diamond rings on his fingers, diamond tie-pin and silk scarf, and he had a big fat cigar in his mouth, very posh indeed. George wasn't looking where he was going as his eyes were downcast and full of dread. He accidentally bumped into the bookie and nearly knocked him over. Gus caught hold of him to stop himself from falling. "Hey! George, careful there, steady on, you nearly knocked me over then," he said. "What's the matter? Why the long face?" So George told him everything that had happened to him that day. "And to make matters worse," he concluded, "just look what I've done to my shoe on that stupid mat well in your shop." He showed Gus the loose flapping sole of his shoe. Gus said, "Tut! Tut! We can't have that now, can we George? But don't you worry old friend, here let me help you." Then from his pocket he pulled a thick roll of bank notes. The roll of money was about four inches in diameter, there must have been at least £500 in that roll of money, it could very well have been a lot more as it had an elastic band around it holding it all together. George's eyes lit up, he looked heavenwards, clasped his hands together and under his breath he muttered, "Thank you God, thank you for saving me." He pulled Gus towards him and gave him a hug, sobbing, "Thank you! Thank you! Oh Thank you!" He was shaking and rubbing his hands in anticipation. Gus said after he had got his breath back, "Steady on George, there is no need for that." Then he pulled off the elastic band and with a flourish said, "Here you are George, put this elastic round your shoe." George's eyes went red and bulged with a mad gleam, a vein on his neck was clearly visible pulsing away fit to burst, and a white froth appeared at the corner of his mouth. "Grrr! I'm gonna kill yer," he roared, his hands like steel claws reaching out to squeeze the life out of Gus, who screamed in terror and ran into his shop, slamming shut and bolting the doors.

When George finally got home that fateful day, his wife was in the kitchen frying bacon and sausages for his dinner. That's when George made another big mistake, I would venture to suggest it was his biggest mistake. He told her that he had lost all his wages while she still had a heavy skillet of bacon, sausages and hot fat in her hand. And that's how he came by his injuries.

The weeks and months passed quickly. We were working seven days a week and all the overtime we were asked to do. Britain's building trade was booming. One day I was told that Mr. Birtles wanted to see me; could I call into the office on my way home after work? I was feeling a bit nervous wondering what he wanted to see me for. When I entered his office he gestured to a chair and said, "Sit down Kevin." Then when I sat down he said, "I have had good reports from Bob about you, so I have decided to give you your roofer's card. This will entitle you to a rise in your wages. It's a tanner an hour extra (a tanner is six old pennies, two and a half pence in today's money). "If you carry on like this you will soon be a roofer first class." Well that made my day. I went back to work feeling very elated and proud of myself. They're not a bad bunch of blokes these roofers; rough and ready blokes but with hearts of gold, they would give you their last five bob if you needed it. I felt very proud to be one of them.

Whenever a stranger from another trade came on site and spoke to me, even though most of the time I understood what he was saying, one of the lads would always come over and hover around nearby, ready to jump in and help if I needed it. It was all in a protective way, especially by Wilf. He was only a young lad of 16 when I first met him, but he had elected himself my official interpreter and he would keep me informed about what was happening on site. If it was Stan who was near me when some stranger spoke to me, he would say, "Ne'er mind 'im he can't hear ye, what do ye want?" Now that isn't as heartless as it seems, because Stan was almost blind, so I just put up with it.

A Roofer's Life

*Few people are capable of expressing with
equanimity opinions which differ from the
prejudices of their social environment*
Albert Einstein

ONE OF THE most difficult things every deaf person has to
learn as soon as possible is that for your entire life you must be
prepared for bullying, exploitation and discrimination, which
sometimes can come from the most unexpected people. For
some strange reason lots of hearing people seem to think that
deaf people are easy victims. I know that couldn't be further
from the truth and many hearing people have found that
out the hard way. How you deal with that problem is up to
you, but I do know that you cannot take umbrage every time
someone tries to take advantage of you, you must turn a blind
eye most of the time. Sometimes if you are quick enough
with a witty or ironic repartee it is enough to cut them down
to size. Otherwise it is best to just walk away and ignore them
or you will be arguing and fighting every day. You must adjust
if you hope to survive and achieve whatever it is you hope
for. If the world won't adapt itself to fit your needs, then you
must adapt yourself to fit the world. Don't forget that hearing
people far outnumber deaf people, so it really is a hearing
world.

For some reason I never had the feeling of being bullied
or discriminated against in the building trade in those early
days of the 1950s. If I was then I was unaware of it, as being
deaf maybe it just went over my head. I didn't have a hearing
aid in those days because they were too cumbersome to wear

on a building site, and as they say 'Ignorance is bliss'. Maybe it was because we had not long come out of a war and people were tired of trouble and fighting, or maybe I was perceived as harmless and not being a threat to anyone. Maybe it was because there was no bonus system, which meant there was no competition and scrabbling to see who could earn the most money; that came later with the new bonus system. By that time I had gained a reputation as a strong man and the few people who tried it on with me were soon shown the error of their ways. But I do know that many deaf people were being bullied and discriminated against in other jobs, and some years in the future when I had left the roofing trade I was to experience some terrible discrimination, especially when working for Royal Mail, but they were a completely different type of people from those that I worked with in the roofing trade. I'll tell you about that later on in my story.

As the job at Trafford Park was coming to a conclusion, our gang was being split up. A lad named Tommy Muir asked me if I would like to be his mate. I had worked with Tommy a lot on the Trafford Park project and I had found him to be a friendly, amiable man and I had learnt a lot from him, so I had no hesitation in saying that I would like to be his mate as there was still a lot that I could learn from him. Tommy was in his late 30s at that time. He had been a roofer from leaving school as a 14 year old lad and had lots of experience as a roofer and knew all there was to know about the trade, so I was in good hands. Tommy and I worked together for about two years and got on very well. We had jobs all round Greater Manchester and Lancashire, but then one day we were told that a new bonus system was to be tried and our pay would depend on how much work we did. We would get so many hours to do so many yards of roofing, flashings etc.

A new man was sent to work with us and we had to teach him the trade. Then a few weeks later I was called into the office. A new manager had come to take over the management of Ruberoid Roofing. I can't remember his name but I remember that he was a pompous little man, rather like Captain Mainwaring from Dad's Army but not as funny. He had been sent from Newcastle to sort out the Manchester office and establish a new bonus system. He told me that he was terminating my employment with Ruberoid. I wasn't sure that I understood him, so I asked him to repeat. He said that he was giving me one week's notice. I asked why he was doing that when he had just employed a new man to work with Tommy and me. He said that the new man was not deaf and so would fit in better with the other men than I did, so he wouldn't hold them back from earning the bonus. I was taken aback by that remark. I told him that I had been working for Ruberoid Roofing for five years and I thought that I fitted in and got on with the lads very well. He replied that because of my deafness I would hold the other men back and stop them from earning any bonus. He had made his mind up and wasn't going to change it. I said, "You little tw^*t, for that I'm going to give you a good leathering." He ran behind his desk and said that I should be careful of what I do as there were ladies present. I looked round at the other office staff and none of them would look at me, they were all looking at and shuffling the papers on their desks as if they were ashamed to look at me. I told him where he could stick his week's notice, and then I walked out of Ruberoid office for the last time in disgust. In those days, as well as there being no health and safety, there was also no Equal Opportunities Commission. We had to sort out our own problems.

About two days later one of the Ruberoid Roofing lads called Frank came to see me. He said that he and several other men had left too because of this new manager. Then he said that a new roofing company had started up and wanted skilled roofers, would I be interested? Yes of course I would. So the next Monday I started working with Frank for Amalgamated Asphalt. They were a road tarmac firm branching out into the roofing trade. There were six men who were the first roofers for this new firm, George Hussey and his son Johnny, Billy Bryant, Gordon McIntyre, Frank Burgess and me, Kevin Fitzgerald. They later changed their name to Amasco and became very big. They put in tenders and secured some of the biggest roofing jobs in Great Britain.

I remember that for our first job Frank and I were sent to a place in Rochdale where a new school was being built. The material we were to use was called Strammit boards, which was compressed straw covered with building paper, which was very good at insulating the roof. When we had laid them we would cover with three layers of heavy duty felt bonded with hot bitumen to make it watertight. Those Strammit boards measured 8ft x 4ft and 3ins thick and weighed about 200lbs each and we had to cover about 4,000 Square yards. Frank was thinking that we must ask for another man to help us to get those boards up on the roof purlins, but I told him to forget that as there was a new American bonus system in force and it would cut into our bonus if we had another man. It would have had to be split three ways instead of just two, besides I had just been told by Ruberoid's new manager that I would hold "normal" lads back from earning money and I was determined to show that I was as good, if not better, than any hearing person. I knew that I was much stronger than most of them, so once we had got the first three or four boards laid I would carry the others up the ladder and lay them with him and while he was nailing them in place I would be bringing another up, and so we did that for the rest of the week. My legs felt like they had had a very hard work out, but it was well worth it because we had earned £30 each that week. In those days, especially in that very hard winter of 1963, most building workers were laid off. On the roofing side £20 was far above average earnings on most building sites, and here we were earning £30 each. Frank told me that the men from the other trades were nudging each other and pointing at us and saying, "Those two lads there are on £30 a week cor!" Also my legs had a great work out without having to pay any gym fees. The Ruberoid Roofing Company had lost a great worker in me because of some pompous little dictator who didn't know his job, but this new firm was much better anyway as we were earning much more money than we did on Ruberoid.

Round about this time, I would suddenly have attacks of dizziness, the world would suddenly start spinning round and round and I would have to sit down until it had passed. It was caused by some malfunction in the balance mechanism in my ears, and I had my own idea what had triggered it. There could be weeks between attacks, and it always seemed to happen after I had been in deep conversation with someone and trying hard to follow the conversation between several people. Mam took me to the doctor, who made me stand on one leg, then the other. He asked my mam if I had ever had a bang on my head. She told him no, but that I had had meningitis when I was little. He said, "Ah! That's it, here have him take these tablets three times a day, and don't worry, it will pass." That was it. He never even told us what this dizziness was caused by because he probably didn't know. If he had asked me I could have told him it was caused by my trying too hard and straining to follow hearing people's conversations. I decided then to be more relaxed in conversations and if I didn't understand what people were saying then so what! It would be their problem not mine. I had no problem making them understand me, but if they couldn't make me understand them then they were the ones with the problem, I don't see why I should be continually apologising for not hearing what people were saying to me, and whenever I asked them to please repeat, they would roll their eyes impatiently as if they were talking to a halfwit. Well that's what I told myself, so I became more relaxed and laid back. It did eventually pass after a few years and never came back. I think it was the right decision because by then I had learned to relax in company and not to strain by trying to follow the conversation. If I didn't understand what was being said I just let it go over my head. If people had anything important to tell me, then they would find a way to let me know.

I was working on the new telephone exchange being built in Rochdale with Frank, when an attack of giddiness made me sit down. Frank said, "Come on Kev, get up you lazy beggar." I told him what was happening and he gave me a funny look, then he said, "Let's call it a day, come on we will go home now." I had some difficulty getting down the ladder and on the way to the bus stop Frank kept his distance from me as if I was embarrassing him. I'm sure that I looked as if I was drunk. I could have done with some help from Frank but it was not forthcoming. At the bus stop the attack of giddiness became worse and I had to sit down on the wet pavement, further embarrassing Frank, who jumped on the next bus and left me there. After a time the giddiness subsided and I was able to board a bus for home. The next morning, instead of going to work I went to Amasco's office and told them that I couldn't work with Frank any more. The manager said, "No problem, Kev, I wondered when the penny would drop." I was sent to work on another big job.

Not long after I was told that Frank had been sacked. I worked for Amasco for many years and worked on jobs all over England and Wales. The young lad that I had met at Ruberoid Roofing, Wilf Reid, had also joined us on Amasco and worked with me for some years until he emigrated with his wife and children to Australia on the ten pound passage scheme. He told me about it so I went to Australia House in Manchester to make enquiries about working in

Australia too because we had heard that there was a lack of skilled tradesmen in Australia and there was lots of money to be earned. The pen pushers in Australia House, who had welcomed Wilf with open arms, said that I would be unable to go because I was deaf and it was possible that I would be a drag on their welfare system even though I tried in vain to explain that I had never been out of work since leaving school many years ago. That was just another one of the barriers that was constantly being put in front of deaf people in those days. So Wilf and his family went to Australia and earned a fortune and I stayed in rainy old England.

I decided to get one of the tiny behind the ear hearing aids that the NHS had started providing. I thought it may help to level the playing field a bit and give me a better chance. Maybe it would help me to break through the walls and barriers that I was constantly coming up against. I went to the clinic to be fitted with one and I found it to be much better than the massive old one that I had years before. I could hear much better with it, but unfortunately I still couldn't use the telephone, or understand the words of people who were speaking to me unless I was looking at them, although I could hear sounds much clearer, like cars going past, aeroplanes flying over and, best of all, birds singing in springtime. I couldn't, however, tell in which direction the sounds were coming from, and words were still hard to decipher unless I was facing the speaker and could lip read as well.

One time I was sent to a job in Todmorden up in the Pennine hills. It was a mill and we had to take off the old roof and cover and make everything watertight in two weeks because the workers were on their annual fortnight Wakes holiday, which was customary in the Lancashire cotton towns in those years. We had to get the old roof ripped off and the new one on covering the looms before they came back. We had to lodge in a local pub called the Masons' Arms because we had to work all the hours of daylight to get the job done and wouldn't be able to go home until it was finished. Thankfully it was a fine summer and by the time the mill workers came back we had it all covered and watertight and there was just the finishing touches to do so we could relax and take our time. I found that because of the noise of the looms pounding away the other lads couldn't understand what was being said and I was the only one who could understand what the mill workers were saying, so I quickly became one of their favourites. My deafness didn't seem to matter in such a noisy environment as they all spoke very clearly with exaggerated mouth movements and I could understand every word that they were saying. I had to take my hearing aid off every time I went inside the mill as it was far too noisy for me, the noise actually felt painful and I wondered how these hearing people were able to stand such noise. I found out that they were calling me 'Tony' because they said that I looked like Tony Curtis with my hairstyle. Cor! This was the best job I had ever worked on.

The Rochdale Canal ran alongside this mill, and it was the custom to get a few buckets of water from the canal to cool down the boiler when we had finished with it. One sunny afternoon the mill girls were sitting on a wall outside eating their butties and watching us, giving us wolf whistles and catcalls. We were stripped to the waist in the sunshine and strutting our stuff, flexing our muscles and giving them a thrill. One of the lads named Sid picked up a bucket and said, "Kev, hold my hand." As I got hold of his hand he leaned out over the water with the bucket, scooped some water up and pulled it up. I wasn't ready for it and the extra weight was unexpected, so I lost my balance and we both went in the canal. I went in head first and my head went into the mud on the bottom. I came up spitting stinking mud out and spluttering, as I dragged myself up onto the bank I saw that the mill girls were laughing fit to burst. I also saw that my tiny hearing aid was mysteriously lying there on the bank quite safe and dry. I couldn't remember taking it out and putting it on the bank, so I could only surmise that I had instinctively taken it off and put it on the bank as I was falling into the canal. That surely shows how much value I attached to that tiny piece of wire and plastic, and how important that little bit of hearing that I still have was to me.

I worked on many big jobs with some great lads for Amasco. From memory I can name a few jobs, such as Cammell Lairds the shipbuilders on the River Mersey, and Highland House, which was the new tax office built at the bottom of Deansgate near the Cathedral, it was the second highest building in Manchester at the time, nearly as tall as the CIS building. I have a photo somewhere in the attic of myself standing on the parapet of this building, looking down at a tiny Manchester Cathedral and tiny little buses and ant-like people. It's now a hotel, the Deansgate Hilton Hotel. I must find out if it would be suitable or too expensive for a Boston Spa reunion. I also worked on the massive nuclear power station in Cumberland, in Wylfa Bay in Anglesey, the new Civic Centre in my home town, Middleton, now gone to make way for the new Tesco shopping centre, and the Liverpool football stadium at Anfield, and many more that I can't remember. They are lost to my memory in the mists of time. Nowadays, it would be impossible for a deaf man to get a job as a roofer because of the Health and Safety Commission rules, which is a pity because I found it to be a great and interesting job. Maybe I was lucky in that I never had any serious accidents. I found that if I took extra care and didn't take the job too casually, like a lot of the hearing men did, then I was safe.

I was getting a reputation as a sound bloke who knew his job and had no problem getting work at many other roofing firms, such as RM Douglas and also Browns of Preston with Wilf, who had returned to blighty with his family. The word would go round the grapevine where the big jobs were about to start and which firms had won the tender, so Wilf would phone the roofing firms up and get our names down and when it was ready they would get in touch with us, and so we would move from job to job wherever the most money could be earned.

And so the years passed and before I knew it I was in my 50s. Good Heavens! Where have all the years gone, and how could I have got to be so old and not even noticed it. Yet here I was, a wise old man! That old saying, 'Time and Tide await no man' was very true. I had noticed that as the years had rolled past the lads that I used to know had been disappearing one by one; some had become managers or supervisors, some had left to work for themselves, some had left the trade to find easier work in factories, and, dare I say, some had been killed on the job. You must understand that roofing, whether sheeting, cladding, decking out, insulating and felting, slating, tiling, lead work, copper work, etc was a very hard and dangerous job. And it was a young man's trade. Yet here I was in my 50s and still doing it. The reason why I was still working alongside these young lads was because I couldn't use a phone. This was before the minicoms and text phones were invented and it was one of the main reasons, along with being unable to read or write English, why many deaf people were very rarely promoted in their work. So thank you Mr. Alexander Graham Bell, thank you very much for your great invention! The telephone that he invented was a great innovation for hearing people, but not for the deaf, and the irony of it all was that he was trying to make something to enable his wife, who was deaf, to hear better. So the lesson is that nothing is allowed to stand in the way of progress.

When I first started in the roofing trade in 1956, the older men were given easier jobs or the finicky time-consuming jobs, while the younger men did all the humping and heavy work, but now, because of the bonus scheme, I had to work just as hard as the younger men, skill and experience didn't seem to be important any more. Not only that but the managers were putting new lads to work with me and I had to teach them the trade, and if anything went wrong on the job management held me responsible, even if I was nowhere near when it happened. They said that I was older and more experienced and should have told them what to do. These young lads were on the same rate of pay as me, so I asked the management if they would like me to be the supervisor with the higher rate of pay that such a responsible position deserves. They said no, but if I were to see them doing it wrong I must tell them. They probably thought that I should consider myself lucky to have job at all at my age. By that time I must have been the oldest roofer in Manchester still carrying heavy materials up ladders, all the lads from the past who worked with me were either in management, supervisors, working for themselves or out of the roofing trade. In a ten-year period I must have taken on at least four young lads at the management's request and taught them all aspects of roofing. These young lads had then gone on to become managers or supervisors themselves, and here I was, middle-aged Kev, still in the same job.

I was getting a bit disillusioned and some days I felt like packing it in, especially when one day, one of these men whom I had taken under my wing and taught the trade asked me to go into the cabin. Once in there he asked me to explain how the steel decking sheets went on in a very complicated part of the roof, so we got the blueprints out and I explained the procedure to him. Back on the roof he was very self-important, strutting about and shouting to the men, "You do this, you do that, and you Kev do it this way." I had just spent an hour explaining the way it should be done to him, and here he was telling me how to do it in front of all the men. Yes! The roofing trade was beginning to lose its appeal. I suppose it was like that for many hearing people as well as me. I don't know, maybe I was just getting old and hankering for the old days, or maybe the bonus system had changed people. They didn't seem to be as easy-going and carefree as they were in the golden years of the 1950s and 60s.

I had been working away from home for nearly two years and coming home for only one weekend every month and I was getting homesick. I was really missing Diana and the kids, and even Spot the dog. While working for Browns of Preston at the Wylfa nuclear power station at Cemaes Bay in Anglesey, we broke up for the Xmas holidays. When the holiday was over, I couldn't face the prospect of working away from home anymore. I had been working at this place for two years and I had had enough, so I sent a letter to Browns to let them know that I was leaving. These big roofing firms like Browns, Amasco and Douglas got all the big jobs where lots of money could be earned, but most of these jobs were far from home and entailed staying in digs. Not being able to fully join in the chat and banter, and relying on communication only when the others felt like making the effort with me, could be rather lonely and isolating, so at the age of 50 I had had enough and so I had no regrets about leaving.

As I was well known in the roofing trade in Manchester I had no trouble in getting a job with a small family firm in Failsworth, a suburb in Manchester not far from where I lived. The work there was mostly repairing and patching up old buildings that looked like they were ready for the demolition men. The money was rubbish compared to what I had been earning, but I thought it would do until something better came along. I got off to a bad start with the boss's son, though. He seemed to have a permanent sneer on his face.

He was a rather odious young man with a bad attitude, and his eyes were too close together and this gave him a shifty look. Also, he treated the men with contempt; being the boss's son he thought he was better than us. He asked me about my previous jobs and I told him. Then he asked me how many of these houses could I put eaves, ridge caps and flashings round the chimneys on in one day. I weighed up the tumbledown old buildings and they looked like a health and safety nightmare, so I said I could do two a day. He gave me his sneer and said, "Well, I want four a day from you." He said that he had heard about me and how strong I was, so I should be doing the work of two men. I told him that I could do it if he would put up my wages, because unlike the others, I knew what a fair day's work for a fair day's pay was. He stalked off with his face like thunder.

I could see that I wouldn't fit in at this place. I thought that I would give it a couple of weeks to see if it improved. However, a few days later I was called into the office and told that there had been a break-in the previous night and lots of material was stolen. As I was the last one to be employed by them I was the chief suspect. Then the boss said that if I knew who had stolen their gear I must tell him or he would report it to the police. He said that he knew that I was involved because a friend of his had told him that I had phoned offering to sell all the stuff that was stolen. I told him that he should go ahead and phone the police because it was the first thing he should have done when he discovered the break-in and that I was going to see them now, as I didn't take kindly to being accused of being a thief without a shred of proof, and to say that a deaf man had phoned was just showing their ignorance of what deafness was like. This was in the days before minicoms or text phones, so how on earth could a deaf man have phoned his friend offering to sell stolen gear?

As I was leaving the office, the boss ran after me and asked me not to go to the police, which I thought was rather suspicious. Then the son came up to me and, with the sneer, said in front of all the men, "Why don't you just f—k off, hey! Just f—k off." I dropped my tool bag walked up to him and said, "Are you going to f—k me off then sonny?" He wasn't expecting that, I could see the flicker of fear in his eyes and he looked around to find his dad. I had had an abhorrence of bullies from my days at Boston Spa and I was ready to teach this disgusting specimen a lesson he wouldn't forget in a hurry. His dad ran up and said, "Cool it! Cool it!" I was already quite cool, so I told him that he could stick his job as the wages he paid were not worth getting out of bed for, and I didn't have to take insults from him, his son or anybody.

I spent the next couple of years working for myself. I found it a struggle because I was unable to use a phone. I gave a young lad a job as my labourer and he would phone for me when necessary. Then I found that because he was doing the phoning, the people on the other end of the line thought that he was the boss and I was the labourer. The young lad began to believe it too, so that was the end of that. And so I went back to working for someone and got a job with another small firm doing the same kind of work as before. It was better than the other firm in Failsworth. My reputation must have preceded me because the next few years were uneventful, but by now I had had enough of the roofing trade. I thought that I had been very lucky to work for so long at such a dangerous job without having any injuries more serious than a broken ankle and some vertebrae knocked out of place, though I did have a few escapes from serious injury. I thought that if I could start again as a young lad, and considering all the barriers and brick walls that are put in front of deaf people these days and which I never encountered in the 1950s , then

I would certainly do exactly the same again. I had made some fantastic friends in the roofing trade and I have many great memories. Young deaf lads today will never have the chance to experience what I did, but now, at the age of 55, it was time to leave it to the younger lads and find an easier job.

The Royal Mail

I shall tell you a great secret my friend. Do not wait for the last judgment, it takes place every day
Albert Camus

AT THE MIDDLETON Job centre the lady told me that Royal Mail were looking for people to work in the sorting office. She gave me the address to go for the interview and aptitude test. Next day at the interview there were about ten other people there and I was the only deaf man. I explained that I was without an interpreter as I had never used one before, and also I wanted to show that I had little trouble communicating with hearing people by lip reading. What a naive fool I am! The interview consisted of a man asking a few questions and I thought that I had answered the questions with no problem. After that he gave us a paper with some more questions on it. A glance at it told me that I would have no problem answering these questions either. When we had finished the man gathered up the papers and told us to go home and phone in the next day for the results. I was confident that I had passed as the questions were so easy.

Next day my younger daughter Lynn phoned them for my results and they told her that I had failed the aptitude test. When Lynn told me that I had failed I couldn't believe it, the questions were so easy and I knew that I had answered them correctly. I had no doubts at all about that. The only reason that I could think why they had failed me was that they only wanted stupid people because the job was so boring and mind-numbing that people with a modicum of intelligence would be unable to stick at it. Or, discrimination was rearing its ugly head again.

I had been told that the Equal Opportunities Commission had an office in Manchester Town Hall. I didn't want my kids to think that their dad was a failure, so I went there next day and explained to the nice lady behind the desk what had happened to me at Royal Mail. She gave me an encouraging smile and said, "Leave it with me." Then she picked up the phone, dialled a number and after a few words were spoken she put it down again, stuck up her thumb and said with a smile, "They said that they had made a mistake. You can start tomorrow on the evening shift 6pm to 10pm." I was later told by some deaf people that they couldn't use the equal opportunities people because as part of their own policy of giving work to disabled people there was a blind lady on the reception desk, and when they approached her they were unable to communicate. She couldn't see their signs or written notes and they couldn't hear her voice. I was lucky to go there when it was this blind lady's day off.

So, as you can see, deafness is the most misunderstood and ignored handicap of all and that is just because there is no visible sign to show that a person is deaf. Profoundly deaf people don't wear hearing aids as they are no help to them. When I went to the sorting office on Newton Street the next day, I noticed that all ten of the other people who were at the interview/aptitude test with me were there. So that meant that I, the only deaf man there, was meeting with discrimination that could only be because of my deafness, and that was before I had even started working for Royal Mail. Was I the only one who didn't think that my deafness was a problem? I wondered if the queen knew what was going on at this place that carries the Royal Seal of Approval. What happened at that interview should have been a warning of what was in store for me at that place.

Next a man took all us new workers on a tour of the building, explaining what happens in each section. Most of it went over my head of course, but I could pick up enough information whenever his face was turned towards me to be able to follow the gist of what he was saying. At first when I couldn't understand what he was saying I asked him if he could repeat. He would look heavenwards, roll his eyes and shake his head impatiently, so after that I thought it best to keep quiet. Next we went into the lecture room where an official-looking man with a clipboard spent the next two hours talking about the job and what we would be doing. Seated on my right side was a young black man who kept giving me quizzical looks. Then, after a while, he nudged me with his elbow and pointed to my hearing aid. He mouthed the words, "Are you deaf, can you follow this lecture?" I nodded my head to say I was deaf and indicated that I didn't know what the lecturer was talking about. This man, whom I later learned was named Nicky, raised his hand and stood up. He told the lecturer, "This gentleman here is deaf and he is missing all this information." The lecturer looked flustered like he didn't know what to do, and, after giving it some thought, he said, "When the class is finished I will have a one to one conversation with you, sir. Is that alright?"

I was feeling uncomfortable with all the attention I was attracting, all the other people were staring at me and it had been a very long time since I had been made to feel that my deafness was a problem. Now the attitude of these people was underlining the fact that I was different from them and so I had a problem, but the problem wasn't my deafness but their attitude towards me. Also, it was the first time that anybody had ever called me a gentleman or sir and it made me feel uncomfortable, like I knew they didn't really mean it as I had been treated as an inferior for so long. So I just nodded my head.

When the lecture was over I had to stay behind while the others went for a cup of tea. The lecturer sat next to me and told me in ten minutes what he had taken over two hours to explain to the hearing people. Does that mean that I am far more intelligent than the hearing people and don't need as much information, or did he think that I was a waste of time? I am sure this has happened to many deaf people, so they know just how frustrated it can make you feel.

We had to have another test before we could be taken on as permanent, temporary, part time sorters, whatever that meant. I thought they had some strange customs at Royal Mail. For the next test we had to sit at the sorting table and correctly sort 500 letters. So there I was at the sorting table with a pile of letters in front of me. I noticed that if any of the others didn't know which cubbyhole to put a letter, they just put it to one side, so I did the same. Thanks to my travels in the roofing trade I knew a lot of the places, so I just took my time and made sure it was right before I put it in the appropriate cubbyhole. I reasoned that accuracy was more important than speed. Some of the people on either side of me were even stopping and asking me if I knew where such and such a letter went, and hese were hearing people, supposedly more employable than me. They had the advantage of the full two-hour lecture and the tour of the workplace that just went over my head, so it seemed that all the talking and lectures just went over their heads too.

Suddenly the supervisor called, "Stop sorting, your 20 minutes are up." I asked the lady beside me what was going on? She said that we had to sort 500 letters in 20 minutes. That was the first I knew that there was a time limit on the sorting test. I called the supervisor over and explained that I wasn't told there was a time limit. He said, "I told everybody, so don't try to wriggle out of it, I've got my eyes on you." I asked him: "You knew that I was deaf, did you not think that because I was deaf then I might not be able to hear you? It would have been a simple matter of facing me when you told the others, I would have known what you said, and they would still have heard you." He replied: "It doesn't matter, you will have another two tests in the next few days, it will give you a chance to build up your speed." He counted the letters that I had sorted and there were about 300 and he said that was very good and I should do 500 in the next test if I just discarded any letters that I was unsure of; speed was more important than accuracy.

I was in an alien environment here at the Royal Mail sorting office and wondered if I would be able to stick it. They were making it appear that I couldn't manage without an interpreter. I had managed without an interpreter all my working life, so if they wanted one it would be for their benefit, not mine. Anyway, I resolved to give it a go and try my best. I wondered if I was the only person there who couldn't wait to get to 65 years of age and retire from the rat race.

I was put to work sorting letters at what was called 'The Wailing Wall', two long tables and rows of cubbyholes. There were another two men working there and one of them was Nicky, who had spoken up for me in the lecture room. All the others were women, lots of women. I thought to myself, "Bloody hell Kev! Better watch your language here." It was a big change for me after working in such a strong male-orientated job like roofing for so many years, then to be dropped into this place with so many women. No spitting or swearing here Kev! I soon found out that some of the women could put a navvy to shame with their swearing. It didn't take me long to get used to it because I'm very flexible and accommodating.

One day, well evening, because we were on the evening shift, a man came round. He was carrying a clipboard and speaking to the people on the Wailing Wall and making a mark on his clipboard after speaking to each one. When he came to me he just walked past me and carried on asking the others whatever it was until he came to two deaf ladies, who were also working on the Wailing Wall. He went past them too without stopping and carried on at the other side. Out of curiosity I asked the lady on my left side what it was about. She said that a very thick fog had come down and all the transport services had stopped running, and was asking everybody if they needed a lift home by Royal Mail's vans. I said that he wasn't asking everybody, so I went after him, caught up with him and asked him why didn't he ask me or the two deaf ladies if we needed a lift. He looked at me belligerently, then he said, "Well, do you need a lift or what?" I replied, "No, I don't, but you didn't know that. What about the two deaf ladies?" He said he had asked them and they didn't need a lift, so what was my problem. I replied, "You're my problem. I was watching you and you by-passed them just like you by-passed me. You never asked them, so shall we do it now, come on. So reluctantly he came back with me and asked the two deaf ladies if they needed a lift home because of the fog. One of them said, "No, thanks, my husband always comes for me" and the other said, "Yes, please" as she lived in Failsworth and she couldn't possibly walk that far in the fog. So all's well that ends well, except I suspect that is when I got a reputation as a troublemaker. Too bad!

I asked those two deaf ladies if they had any problem at their interview with the aptitude test. They said that there were no problems as they were accompanied by a social worker who did the talking and answered all the questions for them. So it seemed that because I was trying to show some independence, I was rejected. Maybe they thought I was trying to reach above my status, becoming 'uppity' so to speak, and needed to be pushed back down to my rightful place in the hierarchy of the place, or maybe they didn't like the way I would look directly at their faces when I was trying to lip read them. I'd been told before that the way I looked at them intimidated some people, or got their backs up, as they thought that I was challenging them. I don't know what else I could have done. From my love of reading I know that in the American southern states in the 1950s and 60s black people were treated very badly by the white people. One black lady, Rosa Parkes, was even jailed for sitting in the part of a bus that was for whites only. How dare she! How double dare she! She was getting 'uppity' and didn't know her place. Must nip that in the bud right away. In that Royal Mail sorting office, I was made to feel just like that black lady must have felt, and I think that many deaf people are being treated in a similar fashion in Britain today.

There were many examples of blatant discrimination at Royal Mail, but luckily for me at first I was only working part-time there on the evening shift. During the day I was doing small roofing work with an old mate, Johnny, who was having a hard time and was happy to help me do some repairing jobs.

I had noticed that a lad was always stalking one of the deaf girls and making sexual gestures to her. She kept telling him to go away, but he kept coming back to her and she looked really fed up with him, and while she was sat at her sorting table she would keep looking round nervously to make sure that he was nowhere near her. One day when I was talking to her I asked her about this lad. She said she was really fed up with him and that she had a boyfriend to whom she was engaged so she didn't want him bothering her. I told her to tell the manager and that he would put a stop to it. She said that she didn't want to cause any trouble, but if it would stop him she would if I would come with her to him. As they were unable to speak I was elected spokesperson for the deaf people at Royal Mail. I didn't mind at all, in fact I quite enjoyed it. So I accompanied her to the manager's office and told him what she was telling me. He gave me a cold stare and said this boy was only having a bit of fun, that he had worked for Royal Mail for a long time and he was a good lad, and I should stop putting words into this girl's mouth. I found that attitude unbelievable and it made me realise that all the time I had been in the roofing trade, where we would sort out our own problems in our own way, deaf people, because they had to rely on people in authority to make sure they were treated fairly, had been suffering such blatant discrimination for years in places like this.

So this lad carried on harassing this deaf girl, until one day I saw him going into the toilets. On an impulse I picked up a magazine, rolled it up and followed him. In the toilet. I stood alongside him and as we were both having a pee I said to him, "G----e (the deaf girl) says that you like sex. He looked at me and nodded, so I said, "OK, drop your trousers and I'll stick this magazine up your bum." He gave me an uneasy smile as if he wasn't sure what I meant, so I said, "Come on, hurry up, drop them, I've not got all day." Then he gave me a frightened look and just dashed out without even bothering to do his fly up. He never bothered the deaf girl again.

Another time I was talking to a lady when a man just butted in. He came between me and this lady with his back towards me and began chatting to her. He completely disregarded me, so I tapped him on his shoulder and said, "Excuse me, I was talking before you so rudely butted in", or words to that affect; I may have been a bit more earthy than that if I'm honest. He turned round with a disdainful look on his face and said, "Tell you what feller, if you don't like it, I'll meet you outside after work and we can sort it then." I replied, "OK, I look forward to it." After work I looked for him, but he was nowhere to be seen. I waited for a while then gave up, got in my car and went home. He avoided me at work for the next few weeks, keeping well out of my way. Another man used to come up to me and show me his clenched fist and say, "One blow; that's all it would take for me to flatten you. I used to be a boxer and a man's size makes no difference, just one blow."

As far as I could see these people never talked or acted like that to the other men in the place, so why were they like that with me? I found it very puzzling. I wasn't a very big man, in fact my kids call me 'Little Dad' as I am only 5ft 7in tall and they tower above me. These men had worked at the Royal Mail for a number of years and during that time they had never lifted anything heavier than a letter, so why did they think they were such strong and hard men? The attitudes that I was coming up against seemed to confirm my thoughts that the aptitude test was to select the most stupid people for work at Royal Mail. I was already a marked man with the management because of the stance I was taking against the bullying and discrimination, so I kept quiet (for the time being).

I couldn't understand why these people had such a low opinion of us people with disabilities, or if that bad attitude was just for deaf people whom they mistakenly thought were also 'daft'. I had met such ignorant people before, but not to the extent that these people were, and that is when I began to wonder further if the aptitude test for entry into Royal Mail employ was to sort out the stupid ones for the job as it was so boring and mind-numbing no normal person would be able to stick it for long, and I had somehow unwittingly slipped through the net. Once a man came round with a bucket collecting money. When I asked him what it was for he said that it was for a little girl who needed to be sent to America for an operation to save her life. I noticed that these same people who were so nasty to us deaf workers were giving money very generously. I was very puzzled why they were so different in their attitude to the deaf workers. I read once that people tend to be afraid of what they can't understand, so maybe that is the answer. Anyway, a job was a job. It wasn't hard, just boring. If only I could be able to stick with it until I retired in ten years' time. Ten years. Ten Years! Whoo!! I resolved to try my hardest to keep my temper and not let any of these strange people rile me. Just learn to be patient, Kev. After all, you managed to get through eight years at St John's, Boston Spa when you were just a kid, so this should be like a walk in the park now that you're a man. But these strange (to me) people seemed to be trying to see how far they could push me.

Once one of the deaf girls came to me to ask about something work-related and as we were signing a supervisor came and told her to get back to her station and get working, I pointed out to him that other people were constantly leaving their stations and chatting to their friends and he never bothered them, besides what we were talking about was work-related and as she couldn't communicate with him she was asking me. The silly fool said, "How do I know that it is work related?" I told him that the best way would be for him to go and enrol on a sign language class. The deaf ladies were then forbidden to take their breaks together. When I asked this stupid man why they couldn't have their breaks together, he said, "Because they will sign to each other and nobody will know what they are saying." I couldn't believe it, I had never heard anything so stupid in my life. Most deaf people spend their entire lives not knowing what hearing people around them are saying. I told him that I was going to the Manchester Evening News to tell them this story. Just imagine the headline: 'Deaf ladies at Royal Mail forbidden to sign, while other people all around them are chattering non-stop'. I was sure that the Royal Mail top management in

London wouldn't like it, and so the deaf ladies were allowed to have their breaks together again.

When the time neared for the evening shift to end people would begin getting ready for home. They would begin to put their coats on ready to get off and it was customary for the supervisor to shout, "Alright, you can go now" and people would make a dash for the door, eager to get out of the place. The only way that we deaf people could know if he had shouted was by watching the other people, and when they put their coats on and went out of the door we did the same. We couldn't hear if the supervisor had shouted us off or not, so we just followed the people who could hear. But one day, as I was leaving with all the other people, the supervisor grabbed hold of my arm. As I turned to look at him I saw his face was livid with anger. He was glaring at me and shouting, "I haven't shouted you off yet, get back to work." People were pouring out of the door and he could have stopped any one of those who could hear whether he had called them off or not, but he chose to stop me, a deaf man who couldn't hear. This incident proved to me that I was a marked man with the management. I told him to get his hand off me and I carried on leaving the place. It was beginning to look like my intention to keep a low profile until my retirement was going to become unravelled and I would soon be smacking one of these idiots, so I strengthened my resolve to keep calm and just got on with it, and if one of these supervisors said something funny to me I would just tug my greasy forelock and say, "Yes Sir, No Sir, three bags full Sir" and get on with it.

In the mid 1990s Royal Mail closed down their sorting office in Newton Street in the town centre and moved to a new building situated about half a mile away on Oldham Road. They had all the latest sorting machines and things seemed to be getting better. Unfortunately the attitude towards the deaf workers didn't change, in fact it got worse. Most of the supervisors were people who had been promoted from the shop floor. When working on the shop floor these people were useless, bone idle shirkers, so they had been promoted to get them out of the way and to let the good workers get on with it. This promotion didn't make them more intelligent, they just took their stupidity with them to a more responsible position with more power. They were still morally bereft.

I was now on the night shift and there were still many, many incidents of blatant discrimination. By now I had learned to let most of them go right over my head and ignore them, otherwise I would soon be a nervous wreck. One time I was talking to one of the deaf ladies who was also on the night shift. The supervisor was chatting to a beautiful redhead some yards away and when he saw us signing he came over and told me to get back to my station and work. I pointed out that there was a group of black men who were standing some yards away and had been chatting for half an hour and not working. Why doesn't he tell them to get back to their stations and work? He said, "Never mind them, I'm telling you, get back to your station and work now." I said: "You yourself were chatting to that woman over there and those black men have been chatting for the past hour, what's your problem with deaf people?" He answered: "Don't be cheeky, get back to work." I thought: "I'm old enough to be this man's dad and he is telling me not to be cheeky." Instead of going back, I went over to the black men and joined in the talk with them. The supervisor had a face of thunder as he stalked off, so I had made another enemy. It didn't worry me one little bit, bring 'em on! I asked one of the black men why they were allowed to talk and we weren't. He laughed and said, "If you don't like it, why don't you write a letter of complaint, and see where that gets you." So the management were afraid of seeming to be racists and these people were taking full advantage of it.

I asked Terry Riley from the Deaf TV programme 'See Hear' to come and film the deaf workers at Royal Mail, and to ask them if they were happy or if they had any problems working there. Royal Mail refused to allow the 'See Hear' team in to film the deaf workers, but they still came and we filmed outside the building in front of the Royal Mail logo. When I and another deaf person from Royal Mail had finished signing about all the bullying and discrimination that was going on in the place, the cameraman panned up to the upper floor where a group of managers were looking at us through a window and frowning, but they didn't do anything. We were on a public road, and they didn't know sign language, so for all they knew I might have been praising Royal Mail (very unlikely). A few weeks later I met a deaf man who I will call 'J'. He proudly told me that the Royal National Institute for the Deaf (RNID) had arranged for him to meet the top Royal Mail executives in London. They had a very posh meal and talked about J wearing Royal Mail's uniform while they would film him signing about how happy he was working for them. They must have been getting desperate to silence me. I pointed out to J that he didn't work for Royal Mail so how could he do that. He replied that they would pay him a lot of money and RNID had approved it. I was disgusted and went and informed the union rep about what was going to happen. The Union must have put a stop to that sly scheme because nothing came of it.

Once, when coming back from a tea break with some other men, I was singled out by the supervisor. He beckoned me over to him and when I approached him he tried to talk to me. He had a very bad stutter and I stood there patiently trying to lip read him as he said, "W....w..w.." I could see that he was getting nowhere with what he wanted to say to me, so I took out a pen and piece of paper and asked him to write what he wanted to say on it. He looked angry and knocked the pen out of my hand, so I left him and went back to my work station.

Next day I was given a verbal warning by the manager about my making fun of this supervisor's disability and walking off when a supervisor was talking to me. I found that attitude unbelievable. How can you explain to people like that, but by then I had given up even trying to explain. One day I thought that I should arrange a meeting with the manager of the place and the deaf workers so that we could explain to him what was going on. The meeting was agreed for the following week so that I could arrange for an interpreter. The interpreter that I knew said she couldn't do it as she only worked in the Oldham area, so I went one day to RNID's offices on Oxford Road to arrange for an interpreter. The girl on the reception desk couldn't sign so we had to write our communication on paper. I explained that I worked for Royal Mail and had a meeting the following week with the boss about the bullying of deaf workers and needed an interpreter there to make sure there was no misunderstanding. The receptionist was very evasive and said that it wasn't possible as I had to give them one month's notice if I needed an interpreter, I pleaded with her and told her how important this meeting was for the deaf workers, but she wouldn't change her mind. So I gave up and went home and th next day at work I cancelled the meeting with the boss.

A week or so later, when coming back from a tea break with another group of lads, a supervisor beckoned me to come over to him. He said that I was one minute late coming back from my tea break. I pointed out that the others must be late too. He said, "Never mind them, I'm talking to you not them." I said, "Have I got 'victim' tattooed on my forehead? 'No', then sod off" and carried on to my work place. His face was red with anger as he followed me shouting and gesturing. When I got to my work station he said, "Office now, I want you in the office now." I said, "No, I want an interpreter before I go into the office with you." I thought that after a month the incident would have been forgotten, so I was very surprised to find that an interpreter was there next day. In the ensuing conversation in his office he said that he was going to see to it that I was sacked for disrespecting him and swearing at him. I told him that I had two witnesses who would say that I wasn't late from my tea break and he was the only one who was swearing. He wanted to know who these witnesses were, so I told him that if he took this matter further and he would find out. He dropped the matter there and then, but it had cost Royal Mail about £100, maybe more, just for this idiot to ask me a few silly questions. Luckily he didn't call my bluff, so those long poker sessions on building sites had come in handy. So it seems that deaf people had to give one month's notice if they needed an interpreter from RNID, but hearing people could have one next day. When I read deaf man Doug Alker's book, 'Really Not Interested In The Deaf', I had found many of his comments hard to believe, but not now. I can believe everything he said about RNID in his book.

A few weeks after that incident with the supervisor, there was a very important football match being broadcast on the radio. Manchester United were playing but I forget who the other team was. Everybody was listening to the match and not doing much work. After they had slowly sorted a few letters they would jump up excitedly, waving clenched fists in the air and screaming. Even the supervisor who had made himself my enemy was doing it. I thought, "This isn't fair, I seem to be the only one doing any work." So I went over to the supervisor and asked him if it was true that Royal Mail was an equal opportunity employer. He looked at me apprehensively and nodded his head. "In that case," I said, "I can't hear the football commentary that everyone is listening to. I need someone to stand near me and tell me what's happening because I'm a very keen Manchester United fan and I can't hear it." I could see his eyes darting about as if looking for an escape. Then he said he would have to ask the manager and he went off to consult with him. After a while he came back looking decidedly sheepish. I bet he wished that he had never started picking on me and, hopefully, he would think twice in the future before he picked on a seemingly easy victim.

The period leading up to Christmas is a very busy time at Royal Mail. We were working many hours overtime to make sure that people got their Christmas cards and presents in time. This particular Christmas Eve, as the last card went into its cubbyhole there was a collective sigh of relief. Phew! Another Xmas rush over. At dinner time, which on the night shift was about 1am, one of the lads came to me and said, "All the lads are going for a pint, are you coming Kev?" "Is the Pope a Catholic? Of course I'm coming." The local pub stayed open for the night shift. When we went back to work one hour later, I was called into the office and told that I had blatantly walked off the floor despite the supervisor calling me back. I pointed out that I was deaf and had difficulty hearing if I had been called back, and anyway I wasn't the only one, there were over 30 of us so why was I being singled out? The supervisor said, "Never mind them, I am speaking to you, you have always been a troublemaker." I gave the Nazi salute, clicked my heels, said "Ja, mein Herr" and went back to work with the supervisor following me in a rage, waving her arms about and shouting.

When I got back to my work station a woman at the head of a mob approached me and asked me what I was doing in the office. Was I telling tales? The supervisor was standing beside me, so I told her if she must know to ask her. Nobody was speaking to the supervisor, they were completely disregarding her and she had lost all control of the situation. I could see that this mob were out for blood for some reason. Then the man, who used to be a boxer (so he says), came over. He pushed his face up close to mine, wagged his finger at me and said, "If you..." He didn't say any more because at that precise moment I slipped and accidently banged my head into his face. He fell down squealing like a baby and blood was coming from his mouth where I had accidently knocked some of his teeth loose. The woman who had started the incident was saying, "Oooh! You're in trouble now." I couldn't have cared less. Where was the supervisor anyway? She had very quickly made herself scarce. The mates of the man moaning on the floor made a move towards me, so I turned and faced them with clenched fists and said, "Come on then, I'll sort you Ar£$holes out now." They all hesitated, then stopped advancing on me and sat down again.

Meantime the supervisor had vanished. She had run away and hidden somewhere or I would have sorted her out too. I was in a blind rage, the adrenalin was pumping through my veins. At that moment a lion would not have stood a chance against me. All the years of being bullied, picked on, pushed about and discriminated against had finally brought me to the point where I would happily have put some of these people in hospital. I was 63 years old at the time and these yobs were all in their 30s or younger, but it made no difference. I am usually a very placid fellow. I wouldn't hurt a fly, but they had pushed me too far. I'd had enough of them. I went to the canteen for a cup of tea and to calm down, I felt terrible about what I had done to that man because I am not a violent man, and I have put up with a lot of abuse before and not reacted like that. Over the years I had grown a thick skin as a defence against this type of abuse, so I don't really know exactly what had set me off this night. Maybe because it was Christmas, a time of goodwill to all men, but I wasn't receiving any goodwill from them.

I went searching for the man to make sure that he wasn't seriously hurt. I eventually found him in the toilets where he was washing the blood out of his mouth. I asked him if he was alright, and he showed me a couple of his front teeth that were loose with blood coming from the gums. Then he pleaded with me not to tell anyone what I had done. I just shrugged and said that I wasn't intending to tell anyone. He said, "Thank you, Kev" and then he gave me a hug. Isn't that a weird thing to do to someone who had just put you on the floor? I suppose it wouldn't be something that a thirty-something ex-boxer would like people to know about, that an old man had floored him. Anyway, there were enough witnesses to make sure that the story went round the place without me having to say anything. I had had enough for that night, and as it was already Christmas Day I got into my car and went home before I did some more damage.

On the drive home in the early hours of that Christmas morning of 1998, I couldn't help wondering what had happened to that young lad who had left St John's, Boston Spa so full of insecurities, self-doubt, incredible shyness and a vast inferiority complex. What had caused such a massive change in my character. I certainly wasn't happy with the damage that I had caused to that man that night. I had told them that I slipped and my head had connected to his face, but really it wasn't an accident, I had just reacted instinctively. I don't think they believed me anyway. That innocent young lad who had left St John's in 1951 was a much easier target for bullies, but not anymore, so maybe they will think twice before they try to bully me again. I hope they will as I wouldn't like to go through something like that again.

When I went back to work after the Christmas holiday I didn't know what to expect. Usually at Royal Mail, if there is any violence on the shop floor the perpetrators are dismissed instantly, no excuses. Bullying and discrimination against disabled people seemed to be accepted by both the workers and management, so I went to work expecting to be called into the office and dismissed. I didn't really care what happened as I had had enough and didn't give a hoot what they did. Nothing happened however. The supervisor from that night and all those yobs kept well away from me. They must have known they were in the wrong and so had said nothing. I was toying with the idea of going to them and shouting "Boo!" just to see what would happen, but I decided not to bother. As long as they left me alone I would do the same to them. I hoped that from what had happened that night those people had learned a lesson and wouldn't be in a hurry to pick on some seemingly helpless old deaf person again. Really they were just a bunch of cowardly bullies who wouldn't have lasted five minutes in the roofing trade. I only had another two years before I could retire at 65, so I told myself, "Don't go looking for trouble Kev, keep your nose clean." Then I answered myself: "But I never go looking for trouble, it comes looking for me."

I asked for a transfer to the Middleton Post office. They were looking for postmen for the early morning shift, 5am start and 9am finish. I thought that it sounded good and that it was only half a mile from where I lived. The letters and packages had to be packed in a certain order following the house numbers along the walk. On my postal route there were four blocks of flats as well as other houses, but the trouble began when I couldn't gain access straight away to the blocks of flats. They all had security latches on the ground floor front doors and could only be opened when I had spoken to the security man inside through the intercom. Being deaf, I was unable to answer whatever question the security men were asking. In answer to me saying that I was a postman, asking for entrance I could only hear a faint Buzzz-zzz-zzz, taking that as permission for me to enter. I would push the door but it wouldn't open because for some reason they wouldn't open the doors for me. Maybe it was because I wasn't answering their questions properly. I had to wait until somebody either entered or came out of the buildings, then I could gain entrance. This made me late getting back to the depot every day and the manager was going mad at me for being late. I tried to explain what was happening with the blocks of flats and asked him to put me on a walk where there were just houses, not flats, or get me keys to these flats, or arrange with the caretakers to let me in. The man wouldn't listen to reason. He was so stupid I thought that he must be one of these shop floor workers who had clawed, back-stabbed and pushed others down in his climb up to the manager's job. He said that I was using my deafness as an excuse for being lazy. Sometimes I was coming back two hours after all the other postmen had gone home and he was losing his patience with me, I told him that I was losing patience with him too and was he too stupid to know that deafness means that you can't hear, and I'm afraid that I alsosaid some more nasty things to him. I was sick of always having to apologise for being deaf. Then I told him that I'd had enough of him and asked to be sent back to the Oldham Road depot.

Back at the Oldham Road depot I was minding my own business quietly sorting letters when one of the managers approached me. He said, "Hello Kevin. What are you doing back here?" I explained what had happened with the flats in Middleton and the access problem that I had. He sneered and said, "That's not our fault, we give you a job to do, if you can't do it then that's your problem." I thought, "Oh, flipping heck," or something similar. "Here comes trouble again, will there ever be an end to it?" Ever since I had started working for Royal Mail not a day had passed peacefully. There had always been someone trying it on. I said to him, "You're a really stupid bastard aren't you? Why don't you sod off, go and get some education, then you can come back and talk to me." He gave me a dirty look and walked off without another word and I thought, "That's it Kev, you're in trouble again because you can't keep your mouth shut."

Despite making a promise to myself to keep a low profile until I retired, I thought it would be best to get my attack in before that supervisor, so I broke that promise and went to see one of the union reps. I told him that I wanted to sue Royal Mail for all the discrimination that I had to put up with ever since I had started working for them. The union rep tried to discourage me, saying that if I did that I would, in his words, "F ---k it up for the rest of the lads". What kind of people are they? That was the union rep who was supposed to look out for all the union members, even the deaf ones. I wasn't going to let him stop me. I told him that these lads whom I would f—k it up for were the same ones who were making it very hard for me to work peacefully at Royal Mail, so why did he think I should be worried if I f—k it up for them. I went to the Communication Workers' Union (CWU) offices in Withington on the south side of Manchester. After a short wait one of the CWU's managers agreed to see me. After hearing my story he agreed that Royal Mail had gone too far in the bullying of deaf workers and he said that they would get their solicitors to have a look into my story and see what could be done. After much letter-writing and fax-sending, the solicitors informed me that Royal Mail didn't want the case to go to court, and if I agreed to accept a sum of money and drop my complaint they would see to it that the bullying and discrimination would stop. The union people strongly advised me to accept those terms and, as my aim all along had been to stop the bullying of deaf workers, I agreed.

At this time I was only a few months off retiring. I had been arguing and being a thorn in the side of the establishment at Royal Mail for ten years and I was tired of it. I thought that I had done enough for the deaf cause now and I hoped that in my time at Royal Mail I had sown some seeds of understanding, and I hoped that some other deaf people would benefit from it. But enough is enough, let somebody else take over now. I went to the doctor and told him that I had hurt my back. He was very understanding and put me on sick pay and said that I may as well stay on it until retirement as I had only a few weeks to go. After I had been retired for a number of years I bumped into one of the deaf Royal Mail workers. She told me that after I had left, the bullying had reverted to how it was before.

Green and pleasant land

*It requires a very unusual mind to make
an analysis of the obvious*
Alfred North Whitehead

ON THE ALLOTMENTS where I have a plot, I follow
the methods that I was taught by Mr. Shann, the gardener at
St John's, Boston Spa, when I was ten years old, with a few
additional methods of my own because over the years I have
found that the old-fashioned way suited me best. I would take
advice only if it makes sense to me. One day a man came over
to me, unasked, and tried to show me how to sow beetroots.
He said, 'Kev, you get your line then make a furrow following
the line, then you blah! blah!' I know that many hearing
people connect deafness with daftness, and deaf people do
have an undeserved reputation for being stupid and a bit
slow, but I had been sowing beetroots before this man was
born. I know that I should have felt insulted, but I couldn't
be bothered, things like that seemed to be happening all the
time, so I went into my 'long-suffering patience' mode and
said, "Yeah, Yeah!" and carried on doing it my way. Another
man complained that I never listen to what anybody says.
This man had known me for over 30 years and knew that
I was deaf, and after all that time he still had not twigged
that deaf people cannot hear what other people are saying
and unless they are facing the deaf person he has no way of
knowing what is being said, or even that he is being spoken
to. I have told him that many times, but I may as well have
not bothered. Now, tell me please, am I the strange one, or is
he? Or are these people just looking for an easy target to vent

their own frustrations on. Or what about doctors who arrange phone consultations for deaf patients? This has happened to me a few times. Oh! I could go on. Moan! Moan! Groan! I am becoming paranoid.

Another time, I was digging up the first of the seasons potatoes and I saw some of the men talking heatedly. They had a small pot with a long thin plant in it and seemed to be arguing about it. Then one of them pointed to me and he brought the plant over and asked me if I knew what it was, I took it off him and examined it closely. I'd never seen one like it before so I told him, "I'm buggered if I know." He said, "Are you sure" I answered: "Yes". He took it back off me and said, "That's great, thanks Kev", then shouted to his mates, "Hey Tony, it's an imbugafino." I thought, "Did I say that? I'm sure I didn't say that. What is an 'imbugafino' anyway. Did I lip-read him right? I thought it was very funny and thought, "Let's see how far this goes before the penny drops."

I watched as they talked among themselves, they were scratching their heads and looking puzzled. He then came back and asked me if it was Italian and if it was edible. I told him to plant it and see what it turns out like, then look it up in the gardening book. I have to have a chuckle whenever I think of that incident. It must have been the way I pronounce words, have I still not mastered pronunciation? Surely they were just having a giggle at my expense? If they were, then they were very good actors, but maybe I had just misunderstood them. That's one of the problems deaf people have when trying to understand what a group of people are saying. Whatever it was, I much preferred my interpretation of that conversation because it's much funnier.

On the allotments we have a shop where we sell seeds, fertilisers, compost and all the gardening paraphernalia. We have a rota whereby all must take turns to do duty in the shop. I had no problem dealing with those who I knew, but

I was finding it hard to deal with members of the public as it took me a while to get used to a person's speaking style. I was excused the monthly meetings because the speaking was too fast for me to follow, but I was not excused the shop duty. I wrote a letter to the committee quoting the DDA (Disability Discrimination Act) rules, and asked for another job in the shop, such as filling bags and carrying fertiliser to customers' cars, anything but speaking to members of the public, as this would allow me to do my shop duty on a more equal footing.

I have a very good friend on the allotments and her name is Frances Nelson. She is a nurse and she kindly offered to do my duties on the shop. That was very good of her, so I gladly accepted as I was finding it awkward going sometimes, and at my age I could do without the stress of trying to lip-read strangers who came into the shop. In return I offered to do any jobs that Fran found hard and she asked me if I could put up an arch for her to grow roses on. The next Sunday when I arrived at the allotments, the car park was full. I had a heavy tool bag to carry and could only park down on the road some distance away. One car near the gate on the car park was parked at right angles to all the other cars; it was taking up the room enough for another two cars. I went to find the car owner and asked him if he could park correctly so that I could park nearer the gate as I had a heavy tool bag to carry in. For whatever reason, this man resented me asking what to me was a reasonable request. He became very angry and said to me, "I'll move it later when I'm good and ready, first I am going to make myself a cup of tea, so you can wait." I was surprised by his attitude because he was always nice and sweet to the other people on the allotments, maybe too sweet. About an hour later he came to me and said in a sarcastic way, "I've moved my car now, ok! Are you satisfied now?" I went to find the man who was in charge and who had himself told people to park correctly before. I told him what had happened and he too turned on me and said that I was always causing trouble, and if I wasn't careful I would be kicked off the allotments.

Some weeks later they were trying to get rid of me, even though I was a founder member and had been there for over 30 years. Their excuse was that I was upsetting people. I even had a note pushed through my letterbox by a member of the committee threatening me with legal action if I didn't stop causing trouble. I thought that they didn't want to spend money on making the plots deaf friendly, so if they got rid of me their problem was solved. There had been some pilfering going on at the allotments for some considerable time and now from the hard looks and scowls that I was subject to from some members of the allotment society it looked like, for whatever reason, I was the chief suspect. Being deaf I had no way of knowing what they were saying about me, but body language and facial expressions can tell me a lot. Maybe it was just because I was different from them and that was enough reason for them to suspect me. Thus I decided to go and see the parks and recreation people, who had an office in Middleton and were the people that I first went to when I wanted to have an allotment plot. When I was shown into the office of the man in charge the first words he said to me were, "So you're the troublemaker, I've heard all about you, sbe very careful what you say in these offices." I was shocked at his attitude. He hadn't even heard my side of the story. I found out that a member of the allotments committee had been phoning him and telling him what a nasty man I was.

Then I went to see a councillor for the Middleton area, Mr. Ian Robertson, and he called a meeting with the parks and recreation people and two members of the allotment committee who were trying to get rid of me. My friend Frances was the only other person from the allotments to accompany me and to speak up for me at this tribunal. They came out with all sorts of silly reasons as to why they wanted to get rid of me. There was really no reason why they should. The silliest reason was that I wore a contraption to slyly eavesdrop on what people were saying, as if I was desperate to know what these idiots were saying. I pointed out that I didn't have the slightest interest in what they were saying. I said that it was just a tape player with a neck loop that enabled me to listen to music. I had a smattering of hearing in my right ear, helped by a hearing aid, and I could listen to music through my neck loop, although words from songs were not distinguishable. My hearing aid helped me to hear noises, but not words unless I was looking at the person who was talking, and anyway, if there was such a contraption that could enable me to listen to what people were saying, then I would certainly use it. I didn't understand why they had a problem with that. They could hear what people were saying, so if there was such a contraption that would enable me to hear what people were saying, then why on earth couldn't I use it, why did they object to that?

At St John's Boston Spa I had been brainwashed to think that such people were my superiors merely because they could hear and I couldn't, and here these superior people were making themselves look unbelievably stupid. Councillor Ian Robertson really laid into the committee members. I don't know what was said but his face was red with anger as he was lambasting them and they were looking very sheepish and guilty. The meeting was called to a close with the complainers going off with a flea in their ears. After all that the man who started all this trouble is still there on the allotments. He wasn't threatened with eviction as I was. If the hearing had gone against me I am sure from the attitudes that I was coming up against I would have been kicked off the allotments. There are different rules for people like me. Some days later a cousin came to visit me. She has friends who live near this man. My cousin told me that he was telling all his street about what a nasty man I was. She knew that it wasn't true and she came to see if I was alright. I assured her that I was alright.

There are some riding stables on the opposite side of the path from the allotments, managed by Big Al. Anybody who wanted some horse manure just had to ask him and he would dump a load off for them with his tractor, which had a grabber that could pick up several barrowloads at a time. That is, anybody could have as much as they wanted but me! In all the time that I was a member of those allotments, well over 20 years at that time, he would never dump a load off for me, though I asked him many times. He just ignored me and acted as if I wasn't there, I wasn't important enough for him to bother with. If I wanted some manure then I had to get it myself in a wheelbarrow and that could take the best part of the day to get a reasonable amount. One day I wanted to wheelbarrow some manure from the stables to my plot and there was a car parked on the path. Maybe I could have squeezed through, but with my balance problems why take the risk? I went to find the owner and I asked him to move it as I didn't want to bump into it. He chose to take offence at that simple request and snarled at me, "If you bump into my car it will have been done deliberately", so I had to carefully negotiate around his car with my wheelbarrow.

Another time, as I was digging my plot near the fence, I picked up a piece of leaf. I threw it away and it blew over the fence. Al and another man were standing some yards away. I noticed that Al said something to the other man and pointed at me. That man then whistled and waved his hands to get my attention. When I looked at him he waggled his finger at me and said, "Naughty! Naughty! Don't throw things over the fence." I went over to them and asked this man if he would ask Al if he owned the fence or path. They looked flustered and the man said, "Why don't you ask him yourself?" I said, "Because he is asking you to tell me what to do, instead of telling me himself." Then I turned to big Al and said, "Next time you want to tell me something, be brave and tell me yourself, don't do it through someone else." It is incidents like this that they meant when they said that I was upsetting people. It didn't seem to matter that they were upsetting me; they were talking about me as if I wasn't there.

Those are just two examples of the discrimination that deaf people are facing every day of their lives from bigots such as these. The strange thing about the bad attitudes that I was getting is it only started to get worse after one of the Royal Mail's retired supervisors became an allotment member, the same person who took umbrage when I asked him to park his car properly. I was the one who advised him how to get a plot there. I gave him the phone number of who to contact to get a plot on the allotments, silly me. Whatever the reason they were trying to get rid of me was, they failed. I am still on the allotments and I am not going to be forced off by those people.

Education and the deaf

Self-trust is the essence of heroism
Ralph Waldo Emerson

BECAUSE OF THEIR poor education many deaf people
have a problem reading and writing English, but that does
not mean they are stupid - far from it - a deaf person must be
very clever to cope in a world that is made for people who can
hear. There are many negative-thinking hearing people with
many preconceptions about deaf people. Teachers of the deaf,
social workers etc., who tell us that because of our deafness
we cannot read or write because scientific studies have shown
that our brains are different and cannot grasp the meaning
of words and grammar, they are talking a load of baloney.
Have you ever heard of the saying "In the world of the blind
the man with one eye is King" I think the same principle
applies here. There are many people born deaf who have
taught themselves and now have an excellent command of
English. Those people who say it cannot be done are finding
excuses for their own dismal failure to give deaf children a
good education.

Nobody, no matter who they are, whether they are
scientists or not, can say that they understand how the human
brain works. The human mind has vast untapped potential
and its capabilities are not yet fully understood, it is still in
the process of evolving. These people should be helping the
deaf to think big and have confidence in themselves to make
the best of what they have. The last thing deaf people need
is these people putting negative thoughts into their heads.
I and my deaf friends at Boston Spa had negative thoughts

implanted into our heads from the terrible education we were given. We were told that we must heed our superiors, we must do what we were told and obey our superiors and then we would be alright. We left St John's feeling very inferior to our hearing counterparts. It took a strong act of will, and many years, for me to get rid of those negative thoughts because they had become embedded into my sub-conscious mind. Then I slowly began to realise that I was just as good as, or better intellectually than, most of the hearing people that I knew. I suspect that now I have a 'superiority complex' and that is much better than its opposite, an 'inferiority complex'

Let me repeat, no one person, whether a scientist, 'authority' or whatever knows everything there is to know about deafness and how it affects the human brain, regardless of what some of these 'experts' claim or believe. They do not have the final word on what is best for the deaf and most of them are just quoting from what they have read. In other words, it is much easier to follow what other people have said than to think things through for themselves.

There is a huge diversity among deaf people; no two deaf people are exactly alike in their abilities. Yet there are many 'gurus' out there that will try to convince you that they know what is best for you. This is both an insult to our intelligence and character.

On the 'World's Smartest Website' (http://www.edge.org) I found this review of a book about the adolescent brain by Sarah Jayne Blakemore, with an introduction by Simon Baron-Cohen. I know that it is written with hearing adolescents in mind and not deaf adolescents, but if there was no communication problem between the teacher and deaf pupil then I cannot see any reason why the deaf adolescents cannot learn the English language:

"The idea that the brain is somehow fixed in early childhood, which was an idea that was very strongly believed up until fairly recently, is completely wrong. There is no evidence that the brain is somehow set and can't change after early childhood. In fact, it goes through this very large development throughout adolescence and right into the 20s and 30s, and even after that it's plastic forever, the plasticity is a baseline state, no matter how old you are. That has implications for things like intervention programmes and educational programmes for teenagers.

"Sarah Jayne Blakemore is a leading social neuroscientist of adolescent development. She has reawakened research interest into the puberty period by focusing on social cognition and its neural underpinnings. Part of her question is whether adolescence involves egocentrism, as many popular conceptions suggest, since this is testable.

Part of her originality is to remind us of the remarkable changes in brain structure during adolescence, given the traditional focus of developmental psychology is on early childhood. Using a range of techniques, including using conducting elegant MRI studies, she illuminates a neglected phase of cognitive development. Given that the sex steroid hormones are produced in higher quantities during this period, her research opens up interesting questions about whether the changes in the brain are driven by the endocrine system, or by changing social experience, or an interaction of these factors.

Simon Baron–Cohen, Professor of Developmental Psychopathology and Director of the Autism Research Centre at Cambridge University.

SARAH JAYNE BLAKEMORE is a Royal Society University Research Fellow and Full Professor of Cognitive Neuroscience at the Institute of Cognitive Neuroscience, University College London, UK. Blakemore's research centres on the development of social cognition and executive function in the typically developing adolescent brain, using a variety of behavioral and neuroimaging methods.

On this evidence it seems that scientists are still experimenting on the workings of the human brain. Despite these experiments by renowned scientists we must never forget that no two individuals are exactly alike. We all have our different needs and different paths to follow. Write the following down and pin it up where you can see it every day, have it engraved into your memory:

The Bottom Line
Face it.
NOBODY OWES YOU ANYTHING!
What you achieve, or fail to achieve in your lifetime is directly related to what you do or fail to do.
No one chooses their parents or childhood but can choose their own direction in life.
Everyone has problems and obstacles to overcome but that too is relative to each individual.
NOTHING IS CARVED IN STONE!
You can change anything in your life if you want to badly enough.

Truth be told, you have the right and the ability to decide for yourself what you want to do with your life. This is not to say that you should function in a vacuum, it is always helpful to learn from other established thinkers, especially if they are deaf too, so long as you analyse and supplement the knowledge you acquire from them with your own thoughts and experiences. I am sure that we all know of some deaf person who, after being 'taught' by hearing experts, left their Oral school feeling lost and bewildered in the hearing world and so went to their nearest deaf club where they learned to sign so that they could communicate with their peers and wouldn't be lonely and isolated anymore. For far too many years deaf people have been oppressed, told what to do, and expected to do what hearing people tell them to do i.e. to be led by the hand. There seems to be an erroneous idea among deaf people that RNID (Royal National Institute for the Deaf) is the law concerning deaf issues. RNID is NOT the law. They can give advice and guidance if needed but they are NOT the law.

Some time ago I was in a deaf club and I happened to see two deaf men having an argument. What the argument was about I have long forgotten, but what the argument was about is immaterial, it is how the argument finished that made me give a sigh of despair. The argument went like this: The first man said, 'Yes, it is!' The second man: 'No it isn't!' 'Yes it is!' 'No it isn't!' The first man said, 'Yes it is, and I have proof. See that man over there? He told me and he is hearing, he isn't deaf so he must know.' That shows how many deaf people have been brainwashed to think that they are inferior to the hearing people. Isn't it time that we demanded a better education for our deaf kids so that they can be on an equal footing with hearing kids. Don't let them suffer the same oppression that we deaf people of the lost generations had to endure. We were given false hope, instead of learning to accept, we were told to have pride in our Deafness, some deaf couples were even saying they hoped their children were born deaf. I wonder if a new medicine was invented that could cure deafness entirely, how many of these deaf people would say 'No thank you'

.

Changing Attitudes

If I have seen further than others, it is because I was standing on the shoulders of giants.
Albert Einstein

THE ABOVE QUOTE is a good one to keep in mind if you want to pick the brains of others and change them for your own purposes. What Albert Einstein meant by that quote is that there were many brilliant thinkers who came before him and he could use their ideas. Your mind is like a busy computer, it is working all the time. In fact, it is far more powerful and complicated than any computer ever made, and just like a computer, it is prone to problems from viruses. Its virus is negative thinking, it's anti-virus is positive thinking, so stop messing about with your mind and get positive; change words like 'cannot' or 'impossible'. All negative words can become positive words with just a slight change, so delete the 'not' in 'cannot' so it becomes 'can' and delete the 'im' in 'impossible' so it becomes 'possible'. You don't know what you can do until you try, even if you fail at your first attempt, you have hopefully learned something from that attempt to enable you to try again.

Few of us attain more than 10% of our intellectual or physical potential, it's far easier to just follow the crowd. Most of us live well within our capabilities, and even when the ability to do more or better is there, we don't have the knowledge of how to reach deep down into our subconscious minds and bring it out. It's far easier to just follow the path that the crowd has already made than to blaze a new trail. If everybody is saying the same thing, then it is obvious that not many are thinking for themselves, they are just repeating what they have heard or seen others say. The results of this sheep-like behaviour is what led to the banning of signing in schools in 1880. The dire consequence of not enough people questioning such idiotic thinking by the 'experts' is deaf illiteracy. If there were many literate deaf people before and very few after the change to 'oral' education in 1880, then how can it be caused by anything else but Oralism?

I can't pull any punches on this matter, even if it ruffles a few feathers. We need to move away from the stubbornness and short-sightedness of 'specialists' whose attitude towards deafness revolves around what they have been taught and nothing else. Oralism may be practical for kids who are hard of hearing, but it is useless for profoundly deaf kids. I hope that you can follow the logic of what I am trying to say here. I have never learned much from so-called experts and authorities, rather I have learned most of what I know about sign language and life in general, from the time I was eight years old, from fellow deaf people and reading and writing was taught to me by my sister. I have noticed that many deaf people from Ireland and Scotland have excellent English. Many of these deaf people were taught by finger spelling in enlightened places where the Oralism method had not gained a hold. Now, according to these self-styled 'oral experts' their brains are not supposed to function that way are they? I would love to have this strange phenomenon of good English by finger spelling explained to me convincingly.

In the dark, olden times deaf people were educated by teachers using the Oral System because experts had shown that it was the best way to teach deaf children, so thanks to these 'experts' generations of illiterate deaf people have been produced who think that it is normal for the deaf to be illiterate. These deaf people are the lost generations.

As late as the 1970s so-called medical 'experts' were still giving homosexuals electric shock treatments, or - even worse - lobotomies to 'cure' them (poor Alan Turing). For years scientists have led us to believe that vitamin C was the best thing to guard against the common cold, but now they are saying that vitamin C is useless for colds and to take vitamin D instead, so it seems that these people who are always telling us what to do don't really know what to do themselves. Therefore one must not blindly accept everything these 'experts' tell us as established fact; think about it, question it. Most of them are just following the lessons they learned from their teachers in the past, few of them have ever had an original thought of their own. They are just following the path of popular thinking, as in the bad old days when hearing teachers were blindly following the oral method of teaching deaf kids, as taught to them by the Ewings of Manchester University. Not one of them thought to question it, not one of them thought, 'Hang on a minute, this is not giving good results.' To me it is obvious that you can't solve the problem of deaf illiteracy by using the same thinking and methods of teaching that created it in the first place. I hope that the Oral System has lost all credibility now after more than 100 years of failure. It may be good for teaching parrots to talk, but it does not teach a deaf child how to think. Remember that people who are too weak to follow their own dreams will always try to find a way to discourage yours and make you follow the crowd.

Here is another example of this sheep-like behaviour. Have you noticed how many people are now carrying plastic bottles of water and drinking from it all day? Some 'guru' in the employ of the water bottling industry has stated that to be healthy people must drink at least eight glasses of water a day, preferably bottled water, and that is in addition to your normal cups of tea, coffee, soft drinks and/or milk. If you do drink that much water then you had better not stray too far from a toilet, or carry a portable loo with you. Also you must realise that drinking too much water will flush all the nutrients, vitamins and minerals out of your body. You must also understand that drinking too much water may cause sodium levels in your blood to drop to dangerously low levels, causing hypernatremia, a dangerous condition where your cells swell with too much water, certain harmful chemicals also leach out of the plastic bottles into the water.

Drink when thirsty, when training or working hard and sip water frequently to keep hydrated but don't guzzle it. If your urine is a pale yellow then you are staying well hydrated and have nothing to worry about. We have some of the best and cleanest tap water in the world. Back in the day, when we were thirsty we drank water from the fountain in the park or from the tap at home, despite that we are still alive today. There really is no need for all these plastic bottles of water, many of which have been flown in from abroad. These empty plastic bottles also go to further contaminate our country.

I wonder, does history record any instance in which the majority was right? I very much doubt it as most people were just following the ideas of one or two powerful speakers. You should never accept anybody's arguments based on blind faith. An idea, any idea, regardless of its source should be critically analysed and evaluated for truth and validity before being accepted. Truth can be determined only by sound reasoning and logic. Many established 'truths' in numerous fields are based on false assumptions and false premises. How many credulous people are there who still believe the superstitious dogmas and ridiculous fables they were taught in infancy? As the brilliant author Mark Twain once said: 'Faith is believing in something that a man knows ain't true'. If I had lived 200 or so years ago I would probably have been tortured to make me recant, and then burned at the stake for saying that.

Before 1880 deaf teachers were producing literate deaf kids, then for some unknown reason the hearing authorities banned signing, sacked all the deaf teachers and brought in hearing teachers who were unable to communicate with the deaf children. That was the beginning of the end of deaf literacy, except for a few exceptionally brilliant deaf men, men like Mr. Caproni, who saved many deaf kids from a life of illiteracy, and despite what many hearing people say, you can be both a deaf-born expert signer and fully literate in the English language, just like Mr. Caproni was. Now, over 130 years later, the deaf are just beginning to recover from that idiocy. My mind boggles at the sheer stupidity of it all and I just cannot understand how it was allowed to happen.

A very clever man called Douglas Adams once said: "Human beings, who are almost unique in their ability to learn from the experiences of others, are also remarkable in their apparent disinclination to do so." Does that statement explain why it has taken so long for deaf education to recover from those dark days of oralism? Ignorant people can be dealt with, they can be taught, but stupidity is much harder to deal with because that is genetic, and you cannot do anything about that except ignore these idiots and hope that they will either be found out for what they are or just go away. I fail to see how these professional 'experts' can be respected by the deaf community. Isn't respect supposed to be earned and not just given because of who or what a person is? To show what I mean, here are some bad predictions from some leading experts. These predictions are laughable now in retrospect, but at the time they were made only a handful of people questioned or objected to them. And because of those few people who did question them human progress took a leap forward.

Some Bad predictions:

'There is no reason why anyone would want a computer in their home' - Ken Olsen, an engineer who co-founded the Digital Equipment Corporation (DEC) in 1957.

'While theoretically and technically television may be feasible, commercially and financially it is impossible' – Lee De Forest, famous inventor and one of the fathers of the 'Electronic age'.

'We don't like their sound, and guitar music is on the way out' – The Decca Recording Company, referring to the Beatles in 1962.

'There will never be a bigger aeroplane built' – A Boeing engineer talking about the amazing 247, an all metal twin-engine aeroplane built in 1933 and which held ten people.

Role Models

Nourish your hopes, but do not overlook realities
Sir Winston Churchill

NOW, SHALL WE move on to another topic? One of the greatest role models for people with hearing problems is the amazing Ludwig Van Beethoven. While browsing on the internet one day I stumbled upon his biography, written by a man named Rob Drucker. I found his life story fascinating. Rob had this to say: "It is well known in music circles, and among historians that Ludwig Van Beethoven was one of the greatest composers of all time; no other composer came close to this genius who wrote over 200 musical works."

The most magical of all symphonies was his famous fifth. Though the Fifth Symphony is his most popular composition, Erioca, his Third Symphony, was his most triumphant. This Symphony was written between 1803 and 1804 after the composer had become deaf, and it changed 18th century musical ideas forever. It brought a new and heightened power of orchestral sound, never before had any audience heard music so magical in artistic scope and structure.

Beethoven had originally composed his third Symphony as a musical score about Napoleon Bonaparte, whom the composer had greatly admired, he even referred to his new work as 'Bonaparte', but not for long. After the Bonaparte Symphony was completed, Beethoven re-titled his new composition in disgust after hearing news that Napoleon had proclaimed himself 'Emperor' of France. This news sickened Beethoven and it opened his eyes to see Napoleon in a different light as a ruthless, power-seeking, and dangerous egomaniac. Beethoven was distraught that he had written such a grand symphony about a man whom he now saw had become a dictator and tyrant, so he changed the name of the Bonaparte Symphony to 'Heroic Symphony', composed to celebrate the memory of a great man, an anonymous man.

Although Beethoven changed the name of his great work, he did not change even one single musical note. This suggests that Beethoven's third Symphony was really about his own ideals, and not about Napoleon. To really understand and appreciate the true meaning of Beethoven's Heroic Symphony one must realise that in 1802, at 31 years of age, the composer became deaf. Try to imagine it; here he was, just beginning to make his mark as a virtuoso composer and he loses the ability to hear his own music played. What a tragedy it seemed to all the people who knew him.

At first his loss of hearing caused the composer such inward defeat and despair that he seriously thought of suicide as the only way of coping with such a devastating loss. In a letter to his two brothers the composer wrote: "What a humiliation when people standing either side of me can hear at a distance a flute being played, and I cannot hear it, or hear the singing of a shepherd and I cannot hear a sound, such circumstances brought me to the brink of despair and had well-nigh made me put an end to my life."

While the onset of deafness had caused what seemed to be a formidable struggle for Beethoven, he slowly came to realise that the only thing that was thwarting his musical talent was his apparent willingness to give it up, not his hearing loss. In his letter to his brothers Beethoven stated: "Ah! It seemed to me to be impossible to quit the world before I had produced all that I felt myself called upon to accomplish." This realisation was a big turning point for the young and deaf composer, and it was one that made his Third Symphony, one of the greatest compositions in the history of music, come alive. By putting his head down onto his piano and feeling the vibrations through his incisor tooth, which he placed on the piano, he was able to compose. That is showing truly amazing positive thinking. What an amazing role model for any disabled person, not just deaf people.

Ludwig Van Beethoven's story should have each and every one of us taking a fresh, new, clear look at what we perceive to be handicaps in our lives. We all face seemingly insurmountable obstacles from time to time, but many times these obstacles can be overcome by simply changing the way we think. A loss can be turned into a triumph by strengthening those senses that we still have, and by creating new pathways to success. Beethoven's Erioca surely will tell us that this is indeed true. How else can you explain that a musical masterpiece was created by a person who could not hear one note of his own music being played?

Now go and put the kettle on, make yourself a nice cup of tea, get the choccy biscuits out, sit down, and think about Ludwig Van Beethoven for a few minutes, and marvel at the resilience of the human spirit. Just think for a moment, if things come too easy for you the 'fight' that is in each and every one of us is rarely stirred enough to thrust us into action. Hardship and struggle during the formative years of your life can light a fire within you like nothing else. So maybe I should be giving thanks to St John's, Boston Spa, after all.

Another famous Deaf artist was Francisco De goya. De Goya was born in 1746 at Fuendetados Spain and died in 1828 in Bordeaux France. He was an innovative Spanish romantic painter to be mentioned in the same class as El Greco and Diego Valezquez and other great Spanish masters.

Francisco De Goya was a genius in a very different way that Beethoven was. Goya's art medium was painting while Beethoven's art was musical composition. Goya was originally trained in the rococo style, but later he transformed his style and created works that have as great an impact today as when they were created. Goya has been regarded both as the last of the old masters and the first of the moderns. Both men were deaf but their cases were not comparable for whereas Goya flourished in the visual art of painting, Beethoven had to overcome his lack of hearing in the auditory field of music.

Goya's deafness changed him from a conventional court painter into an inventive, novel genius giving out a torrent of works coming from his tormented inner self; indeed some of his works were very macabre and dealt with the executions of Spanish soldiers by French troops. By contrast Beethoven, already an established composer before he became deaf could not exploit his deafness, but had to use his knowledge and memory to get around its limitations in the world of sound and music.

Given these conflicting conditions, it becomes an immense problem to decide which of them deserves the honour of overcoming adversity the most. Much of the problem concerns the differing natures of auditory and visual perceptions. We deaf people may perceive the arts of music and painting differently, we are more likely to think that deafness would not hold a painter back, in fact rather than be a hindrance being deaf would be a positive benefit to a painter, it would enable him to concentrate better and to give his entire attention to his paintings with no fear of being distracted by any background noises.

But; the effect of deafness on music (auditory) and painting (visual) differs fundamentally, thus Beethoven had a mountain of adversity to overcome while Goya was not handicapped in the least by auditory lack in the visual world of painting.

Very often with the onset of deafness at whatever age it is usually accompanied with feelings of inferiority. Many times these feelings of inferiority can inhibit someone's chances of developing their capabilities and aptitudes. Often these feelings of inferiority can make a person give up before they have even put up a fight because they are overwhelmed by real or imaginary shortcomings.

Once the sense of inferiority, whatever the reason for it may be, once it has become a part of their personality, if they don't want to just roll over and give up, then the fight is on. The individual must compensate for those feelings and once the person can accept that he has an inferiority complex he can take control of the direction and method of compensation.

The most common compensation is the development of an attitude of superiority. Most people who at first glance radiate with self-assurance are only putting on a defence to protect their feelings of inferiority, we all know of deaf people who are always boasting about their jobs and how much money they earn, how clever their university educated children are etc. They should be very careful not to over compensate

Another way to counter these feelings of inferiority is to fantasise. Day dreams and wishes are fantasies, playing about with ideas and dreams in your head to compensate for an inferiority complex. I wonder, is it possible that this is the secret of Beethoven's success as a music composer and Goya's success as a painter.

If you are a deaf person, has this little story given you more confidence and determination to push yourself a bit harder? If you are a hearing person, or teacher of deaf children, do you still think that deaf kids cannot be taught to read and write English grammar, the language of the country of their birth? If you still do, then shame on you. Maybe the time has come to get back to pre-1880 levels of literacy for deaf kids. I would love to be proved wrong, but I doubt very much if the teaching methods have improved much over the years, improved modern technology such as hearing aids and cochlear implants is the reason why many deaf children are better educated than the children of my era.

A few years ago I was asked to give a speech to a group of people from the education authorities at Rochdale Town Hall. While I signed my speech, one of my sign language pupils acted as my interpreter. Here is the content of that speech.

The Education of Deaf Children

Previous to the international education conference held in Milan in 1880, deaf teachers in deaf schools were turning out well-educated deaf children whose signing followed the spoken and written word; the education of deaf children started on its downward spiral at the Milan Deaf Educational Conference of 1880. There were no deaf people invited to that infamous conference to give their point of view. It was decided there at that conference that deaf teachers and sign language should be banned from deaf schools; that decision is the cause of the bad grammar used in BSL. Since that time over 130 years ago deaf children have not had a fair deal, their education has been abysmal, many are leaving school at age 16 with a learning age of a hearing eight-year-old child. There are many who never catch up and spend a life being illiterate and that is a tragedy.

Then integration was introduced, and because of this most of the special schools for deaf children have been closed. About 97% of our deaf children are in mainstream schools, and still most of them are leaving with the reading and writing skills of a hearing eight-year-old (if they are lucky) no improvement in over 130 years; the professional "Educational experts" can and do argue about the benefits of mainstreaming, and they can appear to be quite intelligent people when they argue for it, but they can offer no plausible explanation as to why the literacy level among Deaf school leavers is still so low. If they were to ask any reasonably intelligent Deaf adult, they would soon learn why.

Many Deaf children find it a hard struggle in mainstream schools where the level of communication support is very poor and bullying by the hearing children is rife; special schools for deaf children are needed, with teachers and staff who are deaf themselves, they should be well educated and qualified; these very special people are going to be very hard to find because of the literacy level of deaf school leavers; there is also a rule that any teachers of deaf children must first teach hearing children for 2 years before they can teach deaf children, thus making it impossible for a deaf person to become a teacher of deaf children. I am not sure if this rule still applies, all I know for sure is that every time I have tried to improve my life in the past I have come up against brick walls and barriers such as this.

The birth of a baby is a wonderfully happy time for most parents; their lineage will be carried on. Most parents want a better life for their children than they had themselves, so the child's future will be excitedly planned. If the child is born Deaf then these great plans are dashed depending on whether the parents are hearing or deaf. Hearing parents and their deaf child usually have a very hard and painful time, maybe the parents have never met deaf people before so they are shocked and may spend years dragging their deaf child around to see the specialists who usually have negative views on deafness and look upon it as a defect and will advise them that their deaf child will need otologists, audiologists, speech therapists, special education etc. These hearing parents don't know that other parents, deaf parents, raise their deaf children successfully without many of these services, they raise their deaf children more successfully than hearing parents who use these services a lot. judging by the results of psychological and learning tests. Most deaf children of deaf parents function better than deaf children of hearing parents in all learning, linguistic and social areas, from infancy they are not treated as if they are defective or handicapped, but as normal members of a normal family. In the past some deaf children of deaf parents did not realize that there were hearing people in the world who communicated in a strange way by moving their mouths until they were of school age (Look up ''Martha's Vineyard' on the internet)

Deaf children of deaf parents, like any other children can grow up to become adults with a strong sense of who they are and a positive view of their ability to do what they want to do, and not the hearing worlds negative view of their abilities. There is another way by which the functioning of the deaf home and the role of sign language in the development of their children can be viewed. 90% of the children of deaf parents are hearing. These children of deaf parents very often function bilingually using both sign language and spoken English with ease. Many of them have parents who have had a very poor education and very poor paying jobs, nevertheless a lot of these hearing children of deaf parents grow up to be very clever people indeed and many enter the professions.

Deaf teachers have not taught deaf children since 1880. Nowadays Deaf people like me teach hearing people how to sign so that they can sign to the deaf children, but they will never know what it is to be deaf. A deaf teacher with his superior signing skills would be able to get inside deaf children and draw them out, and put knowledge there; a good deaf teacher will also be a good role model for the deaf children. This discrimination that messes up our deaf kid's education must be stopped now, and deaf children must be put on an equal footing with their hearing school friends.

Because of their deafness and poor education the deaf are a very vulnerable part of our society, so often they cannot read or write in any plausible way, because of this they don't have the communication skills to argue their own case. They have to rely on politicians and other people to highlight their cause, but they are so often let down by them, and because of their illiteracy and inability to communicate with hearing people they have to rely heavily upon interpreters; have you noticed how much interpreters are charging for their services nowadays? It's no wonder they don't want a better education for the deaf and are pushing B S L and its silly grammar for all they are worth.

There are many deaf people, who try to help themselves, but they do not always have the skills to do this of their own volition; when people cannot fight their own battles then their fate depends on the rest of society. Do enough people want to help them, without wanting to take over and control their lives?

Over the years many people have joined my sign language classes with the sole aim of earning as much money as they can from the plight of the deaf. Surely with the proper education focused mainly on learning the English language and communication skills many deaf people would have no need to rely on these people. At first my speech was met with silence then there was a deafening (Whoops!) applause. But nothing was done about it, none of those people came to me afterwards to ask questions or talk about that speech. ; it was almost as if they were afraid to try to communicate with me, probably the mad gleam in my eyes put them off (joke) maybe it will take a few years for the seed that I sowed to germinate.

By a strange coincidence, and despite being one of the most successful sign language classes in the area and having been a tutor for over 10 years, not long after giving this speech, I was told that my services were no longer wanted despite my classes having glowing reports from the Ofsted inspectors, I often had up to 25 students in my classes and many of them were very upset at not being allowed to finish their courses. They signed a petition, but to no avail. I was told that it was because of government cuts, yet many other courses such as flower arranging, French,Italian and Spanish languages were kept on, does that mean that things like flower arranging etc are more important than being able to communicate with Deaf people? Or does it mean that sign classes are too expensive compared to other language classes?

I derived the title of my first book "Deafness of the mind" from a quote by the brilliant author Victor Hugo, here is another of his quotes: "There is one thing stronger than all the armies in the world: and that is an idea whose time has come." I can almost believe that he had deaf people in mind when he wrote that.I must remind myself to research the life of Victor Hugo to see if I can find any connection he may have to deaf people as he seems to be very understanding and insightful to the problems that many deaf people have in the hearing world.

Perhaps when we have more educated deaf people we can get back our deaf teachers for deaf children. Not all deaf children can take advantage of modern technology; there will always be some deaf kids whom hearing aids and cochlear implants cannot help. These are the children who need a deaf adult to be teacher, mentor and role model to help them through the first hurdles that life will put in front of them. Beethoven and Goya would make ideal role models to encourage deaf kids and I am sure there are many more deaf achievers to fill that role too.

With the closure of so many deaf schools today, deaf children need access to their history and culture, they need to be told about what deaf achievers have done in the past so that they can have deaf role models they can read about, look up to and try to emulate. Hearing people don't always understand how important deaf culture is to deaf children. They look upon deafness as a "medical condition, a deficit that must be treated, they don't seem to realise they are sending very negative signals to deaf kids by taking that stance.

When I have taken some of my hearing students to the deaf club to introduce them to deaf people, they are always amazed as they see hands and fingers flying about at lightning speed as the deaf people are deep into conversation, then they realize they are in a different world. This is deaf culture that is so important for deaf people, in such an environment it is the hearing people who are at a disadvantage, and it makes them realize what deaf people have to put up with every day of their lives in the hearing world. We deaf people are unique, we are different from hearing people, but we are in no way inferior to those who can hear, we have our own culture and visual language and that is something to be immensely proud of.

I once read an amazing book written by David J Schwartz called "The Magic of Thinking Big". In this book there is a paragraph that states "Real education, the kind worth investing in, is that which develops and cultivates your mind. How well-educated a person is, is measured by how well his mind is developed'—in other words, by how well he thinks. Anything that improves thinking ability is education, not filling people's minds with negative thoughts. I have also read in a book about the life of Abraham Lincoln where the author says that the former President of the United States of America often sought friends and mentors from people he could learn from, be challenged by and be encouraged by. This was one of Lincoln's secrets for gaining what he called an 'advanced' education and is the reason why despite the fact that he only attended school for a total of about one year during his growing years he was able to become the President of the United States of America.

In today's political climate with this government making deep cuts into education and social services (less interpreters, social workers, etc) surely it would be better for deaf people to strive to become more independent, and the best way to do that is to be better informed and the best way to be better informed is to become more skilled in reading and writing. There are many hearing people who cannot read or write, but unlike deaf people, they can get by with speech and using their hearing ability. As recent events have shown, it is a mistake to think that when hard times come the hearing community will look after the ones with disabilities, we are not all in it together. When cuts have to be made the deaf and other disabled are always the first to suffer, when jobs are scarce the deaf/ disabled are always the first to get the push, no matter how clever or talented they are.

I have gathered much of the information to enable me to write this book because of my reading ability, as BSL has no written language, how can deaf BSL users acquire the knowledge to express their stories in book form. I am sure that there are many deaf people who have very interesting stories to tell, stories that could add many interesting facts to the history of deaf people, but they just don't have the words or grammar to write their stories. Many don't even have the ability to follow the subtitles on films or television.

Many deaf people have a different way of approaching life's problems, they tend to think things out for themselves as they cannot rely on the written or spoken word for advice as they are not sure of the meaning of what they are reading, so many hearing people think that deaf people are strange, or what they call "Odd balls" because they don't follow the established way, they do their own thing.

Because they have not been told how to solve problems, they approach the problems from a different angle that hearing people would, they don't follow the herd, and they go along the road less travelled.

Retirement

Never be satisfied with what you achieve because it pales in comparison with what you are capable of doing in future

Rabbi Nochem Kaplan

AND THAT IS the story of a deaf man's struggle trying to cope and work in the hearing world. You can believe me when I say it was no easy task. I learned a lot from my years working for Royal Mail. For example, I learned how to keep my temper, how to be patient and how to swallow my pride and eat humble pie. I hope that after reading my story you will now realise that there is a lot of unfairness in the world. In the Britain of 2012, the politics of 'F---k you Jack, I'm ok' is still going as strong as ever. After many thousands of years of evolution humankind is still not perfect, but there are hopefully thousands of years more of evolution yet to come for us to do away with envy, greed, cruelty etc., that is if somebody doesn't decide to blow us all up in the meantime. Maybe after a few more decades of evolution, spare part surgery will have been perfected and there will be no more deaf or other disabled people and everybody will be equal and free to worship their religion and live their lives peacefully. I'm sure that God in Heaven is looking down on us and shaking his head in despair as He observes all the wars and killing going on in his name. He must be muttering to himself, "I didn't mean it to be like that." Hopefully my grandchildren will still be alive to see the world finally at peace, but it's very doubtful.

Well now, here we are in the year 2013. It seems amazing how the years have flown. After a life time of graft and toil

Diana and I are really enjoying our golden years. I've been retired for 12 years now and it's wonderful to wake up in the morning knowing that I don't have to face any more bullying and discrimination merely because I am deaf, but I know that there are still many people who think that the deaf are easy targets. Looking back I wonder how on earth did I manage to get through all those years and at the same time keep my temper and not seriously hurt any of those bullies, especially at Royal Mail where bullying and discrimination of the deaf employees seemed to be the norm. I think the experience has made me a much more tolerant man, able to understand better the foibles of the human race.

I don't know about conditions in other countries so I cannot comment about them, but here in Britain it seems to be a national trait to bully and pick on people who are different. I can remember when it was Jewish and Irish people who were reviled, then it was black people and Asians. If you don't believe me then just ask yourself, why was it necessary to bring in the anti-racism laws? Now, as those people are not so easy to target anymore who is left for these pathetic people to vent their poisonous feelings on? They must have someone who they think it will be easy to bully, who it will be easy to blame for everything that goes wrong in their miserable lives. Who can't answer back and defend themselves? Deaf people, of course. At Royal Mail this bullying was going on day after day and it made me think that it must be going on in any other large workplaces where there are a lot of people working together under one roof. The sooner deaf people learn English and so be able to argue their case and stick up for themselves, the better it will be for them. I found that at Royal Mail there were many people who knew what was going on, how the management were bullying their deaf employees. These people may have been good kind people, but none of them did anything to stop the bullying; none of them spoke up for deaf people, so in my eyes they were just as guilty as the perpetrators.

Hey Kev! All that is supposed to be behind you now so get on with enjoying your retirement. I know! I know! I should but it isn't easy to forget after a lifetime of discrimination. Even in retirement they were still trying to bully me on the allotments. Sod it! Let someone else sort all that out now. When I retired in the year 2000 it took me some time to be able to completely relax and forget the past. I carried on with my training in the gym at the bottom of my garden because I didn't want to become fat and lazy as I had seen so many retired men turn out when they didn't stay active, I did get a bit of a beer belly, so I cut down on the beer and while I was at it I cut down on the bread and potatoes as well. And I upped my squatting, and it's worked! Some people when they retire take it easy and play bowls as their only means of exercise. I needed something more strenuous than bowls. I also kept on with the allotment as it got me out of the house and from under Diana's feet and I have always enjoyed working with the soil.

The Bible says that Jesus told his disciples to go forth and multiply, so like a good Christian I have tried my best. Now my family consists of my wife Diana, aged 76 and myself age 78; Our three children, Rosemary aged 52, Lynn aged 48 and John aged 43; Four grandchildren: Carrie aged 35, Martin aged 33, Megan aged 14 and Jack aged 11; And four great-grandchildren: Georgia aged 16, Sydney aged 13, Scarlet aged 10, and Tallulah aged seven. As a family we have had our ups and downs, but there is a lot of love and we look out for each other and help with any problems that may crop up. We are a happy fun-loving family and I consider myself a very lucky man to have such lovely people in my family and I am very proud of them.

And so on this note I will end my odyssey and hope that my story has been some help in spreading better understanding between the deaf and hearing worlds.